The Ethics
of Educational Healthcare
Placements in Low and Middle
Income Countries

Anya Ahmed • James Ackers-Johnson • Helen Louise Ackers

# The Ethics of Educational Healthcare Placements in Low and Middle Income Countries

## First Do No Harm?

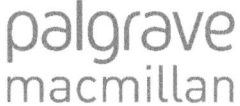

Anya Ahmed
University of Salford
Salford, Lancashire, United Kingdom

James Ackers-Johnson
University of Salford
Salford, Lancashire, United Kingdom

Helen Louise Ackers
University of Salford
Salford, Lancashire, United Kingdom

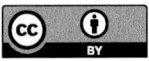

ISBN 978-3-319-48362-7          ISBN 978-3-319-48363-4 (eBook)
DOI 10.1007/978-3-319-48363-4

Library of Congress Control Number: 2017934487

This Palgrave Macmillan imprint is published by Springer Nature
The registered company is Springer International Publishing AG
The registered company address is: Gewerbestrasse 11, 6330 Cham, Switzerland

# ACKNOWLEDGEMENTS

We would like to thank all of those organisations who have supported the development of the Ethical Educational Placements project. The placements could not have been operationalised without the active support of our partner organisation, Knowledge for Change. As authors and project managers, we have received significant support and enthusiasm from the School of Nursing, Midwifery, Social Work and Social Science at the University of Salford. We would like to thank Health Education England (HEE) for the funding we received through the Global Health Exchange (GHE)[1] that enabled us to provide bursaries to students in nursing, midwifery and allied health professions. This support played a major role in enabling us to realise our ethical commitment to widening access to international placements to a cohort of students that previously had little access to such opportunities.[2] The Santander Travel Bursary Scheme also provided important support to students in social policy and environmental and life sciences. Collectively, this support has provided critical time for research and evaluation enabling us to improve and share the EEP model. Salford University has also provided funding for Ms. Natalie Tate to conduct her doctorate in this field (with a focus on

[1] More information on HEE and GHE can be found on their website: www. globalhealthexchange.co.uk
[2] The views expressed are those of the authors, and do not necessarily reflect the views of the University of Salford, Health Education England or the Global Health Exchange

midwifery students). Natalie has contributed significantly to data collection. Ms. Maaike Seekles has played an important role in data analysis. Dr John Chatwin has assisted in the editorial work.

Our gratitude extends to all of the Placement Managers in our partner Universities who have supported the programme. These include: Edge Hill University, Liverpool John Moore's University, Liverpool Hope University, the University of Central Lancashire and the University of Salford.

The Ugandan placements could not have been a success without the support of our Professional Volunteers. We would like to extend particular thanks for the commitment and care shown by Dr Robert Ssekitoleko, Dr Rosie Townsend, Mrs Jean Skeen, Dr Andrew Mullett, Dr Lesley Milne and Mrs Hannah Webster.

We would like to thank all of the 125 undergraduate and postgraduate students who have taken part in placements through Knowledge for Change over the past 24 months and so generously taken part in the evaluation process. They are each and every one a credit to their universities and the UK, and have made a significant contribution to our health system work in Uganda.

Finally, of course, we thank our partners in India and Uganda. In Uganda, we extend particular thanks to Mountains of the Moon University; Kabarole District Health Office; Buhinga Hospital Management; Virika Hospital Management; One Brick at A time (OBAAT); the Kyaninga Children's Development Centre (KCDC) and the Youth and Women's Empowerment Foundation (YAWE). The project could not have been a success in Uganda without the support of K4C's Uganda Placement Manager, Mr Allan Ndawula.

In India, we would like to thank M.S. Ramaiah Memorial Hospital Management, in particular the Departments of Nursing and Medicine, and the Gokula Education Foundation (GEF) for their generous support and assistance in organising the project and providing supervision for the students whilst on their placements. We would also like to thank the nursing student 'buddies' who worked alongside our UK students and assisted them both professionally and socially.

# CONTENTS

# LIST OF FIGURES

# LIST OF TABLES

CHAPTER 1

# Introduction: Why Ethical Educational Placements?

## Globalisation, Internationalisation and Undergraduate Mobilities

Internationalisation has emerged as an increasingly important metric in UK university league tables and marketing. Indeed most, if not all, UK universities now actively promote an 'Internationalisation Strategy' (Coey 2013; De Wit et al. 2008). Much of this development has taken place within the past decade often as a key element of 'marketisation' (Molesworth et al. 2011). This does not imply that universities have not been involved in international relationships for many years; the more prestigious universities have been involved in international activities for over a century. Altbach and Knight (2007) point to a clear relationship between institutional prestige (and by implication resource) and historical engagement with internationalisation processes. Historically, internationalisation has been concerned primarily with research relationships and academic (staff) mobility (see De Wit 2008). In recent years, the internationalisation of education has become more firmly associated with the selling of educational programmes to international fee-paying consumers. The importance of English to these consumers, coupled with the relatively poor linguistic skills of young people in the UK, has influenced mobility flows and shaped the outward mobilities of UK undergraduates. In more recent years, and in some respects linked to the international 'offer', with the intention of making UK courses more relevant and attractive to foreign

© The Author(s) 2017
A. Ahmed et al., *The Ethics of Educational Healthcare Placements in Low and Middle Income Countries*, DOI 10.1007/978-3-319-48363-4_1

consumers, attention has shifted to incorporate an international dimension into teaching. And, linked to this but perhaps rather differently motivated, the broadening of curricula and educational experiences has been viewed as essential to the future employability, resilience, connectedness and culture competence of graduates. Additionally, as evidenced by Health Education England's interest in funding the Ethical Educational Placement (EEP) project, internationalisation has been recognised as a mechanism for accessing new knowledge which students who participate in study and work abroad programmes can bring back to enrich home institutions.

It is difficult to talk about internationalisation without acknowledging and placing it within the context of globalisation (De Wit et al. 2008), and internationalisation and globalisation are often conflated. However, several writers indicate the importance of separating the two concepts. Altbach and Knight (2007) describe globalisation as the wider economic, political and social forces which steer universities towards internationalisation. In this rendering, globalisation can be understood as a set of macrostructures or processes, framing and shaping the internationalisation of the higher education sector: or as the forces which propel higher education towards greater international involvement. In other words, globalisation is an inevitable feature of modern society which has social, economic and political influences and education is becoming increasingly subjected to the wider global economy. On one level then, internationalisation can be seen as universities' responses to globalisation. Equally, internationalisation processes in the university sector reinforce and shape globalisation (De Wit 2008).

Brooks and Waters (2011) add to this complexity arguing that globalisation is itself intrinsically linked to neo-liberalism in the context of increasing marketisation processes. On this basis, they argue that globalisation should be problematised particularly with reference to education. Altbach and Knight (2007) identify three features of the relationship between globalisation and higher education. In the first instance, this concerns the role that universities play in the commodification of programmes. Here, demographic trends are significant with student (consumer) flows showing a marked directional imbalance (from the global South-East to the global North-West). Secondly, the authors point to the rapid emergence of private, for profit universities, particularly in Asia and Latin America. And finally, they refer to new ways of delivering international higher education programmes through e-learning, franchise operations, satellite campuses and split-site arrangements.

Clearly, the global context within which higher education institutions operate is changing and internationalisation comprises an increasingly wide range of initiatives (De Wit 2008). In this environment, recent studies suggest that institutions are not adopting internationalisation strategies in a comprehensive and uniform manner. Further, an emerging body of research questions the compatibility of these marketisation (or neo-liberal) approaches with wider ethical concerns (De Wit 2008). Globalisation tends to concentrate wealth, knowledge and power in resource-rich institutions and international academic mobility favours these systems. As such, and left to its own devices, it compounds global inequalities (Altbach and Knight 2007).

## *Student Mobility*

Student mobilities play an important role in internationalisation and globalisation processes. Until recently, student mobility has not been a major focus in academic research on international migration and population movements, and researchers interested in human mobility, particularly those investigating international migration, have neglected the importance of international student migration (Findlay et al. 2005). This is beginning to change as authors such as Brooks and Waters (2011) and Findlay et al. (2005) have drawn attention to the growth of this phenomenon and the factors involved. Findlay et al suggest that international student mobility is, in part, precipitated by 'rite of passage' aspirations [amongst] young postmodern individuals (2005: XX) rather than factors associated with traditional economic migration. Certainly, the role of travel has become increasingly important in young people's lives fuelled by the promotion of the 'gap year' and other forms of mobility associated with and stimulated by higher education and commercial actors. In society as a whole, the role of travel has increased and student mobility needs to be seen within the context of that wider framework (Brooks and Waters 2011). Indeed, travel for (middle class) young people is now an almost taken for granted part of the life-cycle. Technological developments including mobile phones, Skype, Internet access and social networking have made it much easier and cheaper for young people to spend time away and keep in touch with family and friends reducing the 'discomfort' involved. Spending time overseas is becoming an increasingly attractive (and necessary) 'option' with personal, professional, institutional and societal benefits. The British Council (2013) suggest that international experience is particularly beneficial when competing for future employment and often mobility is seen as a way for graduates to make themselves distinctive and gain a competitive edge in the labour market (Brooks and Waters 2009). Indeed, over the last twenty years the 'gap year' has become a recognised phenomenon (Simpson 2004) and volunteer tourism, something of a rite of passage for growing numbers of young people. Although future employability is a key motivation to travel, mobility also plays a key role in identity development among young people as part of self-exploration and self-development and short-term electives may be important vehicles for this (Brooks and Waters 2009).

In summary, a complexity of processes combine to drive and potentially facilitate international student mobility. At the macro scale these include economic and cultural globalisation and internationalisation of systems. These are complemented by institutional level initiatives and individual motivations including the desire for adventure and future employability.

In March 2012, a Joint Steering Group on Outward Student Mobility[1] submitted a report to David Willetts – the UK's University Minister – making a series of recommendations to encourage outward student mobility. These included:

1. There should be a national strategy for outward student mobility;
2. There is a need for stable funding for mobility for example from philanthropy, scholarships and bursaries;
3. There needs to be flexibility in the curriculum so students can spend time abroad during their studies and for their experience to be more widely recognised;
4. It is necessary to collect available data on mobility and there needs to be some consensus about which data are required in evaluation;
5. Best practice and greater institutional collaboration is needed to deliver greater efficiency and effectiveness and also to increase diversity regarding student mobility; and

---

[1] The Joint Steering Group on Outward Student Mobility was formed in October 2011 at the request of David Willetts, the then Universities minister.

6. There should be a stronger promotion of international electives at school level, at the stage before students enrol at University.[2]

The report also asserts that a national strategy on outward student mobility has the potential to support the widening participation agenda in UK universities[3] by allowing widening participation activities to be integrated into the mobility strategy. The idea here is that that such opportunities should be promoted to less privileged social groups who historically have not participated. At the present time, students who exercise mobility tend to come disproportionately from privileged backgrounds, are relatively wealthy, have some foreign language skills and come from families who have a history of mobility and high educational aspirations. Brooks and Waters (2009) point to the gains to students from international mobility in terms of the acquisition of mobility, social and cultural capital. The concepts of mobility and social 'capital' are of immediate relevance to the current study. Mobility capital is best understood as the benefits accrued from international experiences which translate into enhance employability whereas social capital refers to benefits that travel brings in terms of social networks (Bourdieu and Passeron 1990). Larsen and Jacobsen (2009) argue that even ostensibly touristic activities can have a profound impact on mobility, social capital and future careers. The challenge facing the new generation of educational placement providers is to ensure that access to such career enhancing opportunities are, as far as possible, open to all.

The type of mobility referred to in Altbach and Knight's work (2007) concerns 'whole programme mobility' with students moving to another

---

[2] This is a prime example of how the mobility imperative is being pushed into ever earlier phases of the educational experience with potentially major impacts on equality of opportunity.

[3] Coventry University describes the widening participation agenda as, 'a philosophical position taken by the recent government to re-structure Higher Education and is based upon notions of equality. The aim of this agenda is to offer opportunities to groups within the population, who are under-represented in Higher Education, notably those from socioeconomic groups III-V; people with disabilities; people from specific ethnic minorities'. http://www.jobs.ac.uk/careers-advice/working-in-higher-education/1146/what-you-need-to-know-about-widening-participation

country for an entire degree programme. A second form of mobility is sometimes known as 'in programme mobility', where students undertake short exchanges, usually for taught elements of their programme. In the UK context this is often within the frame of funded European Union mobility schemes dominated by ERASMUS.[4] The final form of mobility involves students who are registered in one country and undertake their taught programme there spending a short period of time on an elective (optional) placement.

## THE 'ELECTIVE'

The 'elective', an optional form of study spent away from a student's Higher Education Institution, usually for a period of 6 to 12 weeks (Banerjee 2010)[5] has historically been – and remains predominantly – a feature of medical education. It is estimated that two-thirds of UK medical students take up electives overseas (Hastings et al. 2014). These typically involve students from high resource settings (such as the UK, US, Canada and Australia) choosing placements in low resource settings. The factors influencing the development of medical electives include a recognition of the diverse communities served by doctors and the need for them to understand these; the desire for students to expand their horizons by learning how other systems operate and the impacts of globalisation (Murdoch-Eaton and Green 2011). Although small in comparison, there are growing numbers of veterinary, nursing (Norton and Marks-Maran 2014), occupational therapy (Horton 2009; Clampin 2008), dentistry, midwifery and social-work students taking up international electives. Yet, in spite of the increase in the take-up of electives across academic disciplines, little attention has been paid to the ethical issues encountered by students and even less consideration has been given to their impact on host countries (Ackerman 2010).

---

[4] The Erasmus scheme was founded in 1987 and provides funding for students to spend a period of their education in other EU member states. Until Erasmus, student mobility was largely individual but once this was established it then became the major route through which students exercised mobility. As part of the scheme students are funded to study in another EU country for between three months to a year. This scheme is widely credited as one of the most successful examples of EU policy. For a detailed discussion of the logistics of whole programme and in-program mobility.

[5] Although this varies across institutions and programmes.

The term 'ethics' refers to the moral principles that govern individual or organisational behaviour. There are thought to be three schools of ethical thought in Western philosophy: first, derived from Aristotle, the virtues of charity, justice and generosity are believed to be dispositions to act in ways that benefit the individual (agent) and the society in which an individual is placed. Second, influenced by Kant, ethics comprise duty, morality, rationality and the imperative to respect other (rational) beings. And, third, the Utilitarian position on ethics is that the guiding principles of conduct should be of the greatest benefit to the greatest number in a society. These schools of thought share a common focus on the moral responsibility of an individual or organisation to act in a manner which does not cause harm to other members in society. The phrase 'First do no Harm' (*Primum non nocere*) is a guiding principle for physicians in their practice and forms part of the Hippocratic Oath, the moral code for ethical conduct and practice in medicine. Derived from this is the principle of 'non-maleficence' (Sharp 1997) which denotes non-harming, or inflicting the least harm possible, to reach a beneficial outcome. For the purposes of this book, we borrow this maxim to frame our focus on undergraduate educational placements, and our examination of the learning and impacts which occur when students from high resource settings spend time in low resource settings as part of their university education. The concept of 'Ethical Educational Placements' raises two broad areas of ethical concern. The first area concerns practice in the sending country; in this case the UK. As noted above; the concept of an 'elective' in the UK has been closely associated with the mobility of medical students, and electives in that context have formed an increasingly important 'rite of passage' amongst this relatively privileged student cohort. This growing 'expectation of mobility' (Ackers and Gill 2007) or 'mobility imperative' (Cox 2008) is also seen in many other disciplines and places increasing pressure on students to build and evidence mobility capital. Although essentially extra-curricular, this experience forms an increasingly critical component of CV-building shaping access to career opportunity. To the extent that international elective placements are just that: namely 'electives' (implying optional choices out with the core curriculum)[6] they raise serious concerns around equality of opportunity.

[6] The University of Notre Dame defines 'An elective course is one chosen by a student from a number of optional subjects or courses in a curriculum, as opposed to a required course which the student must take' (http://firstyear.nd.edu/glossary).

Widening participation to university education in all areas, including medicine, coupled by the extension of this 'expectation' to a wider range of professions where students are less privileged and increasingly debt burdened presents ethical challenges. The Royal College of Midwives National Survey of student midwives (2011) suggests that 70% of student midwives reported having dependents; 70% earned less than £24,000 prior to entry into the programme; 73% anticipated accruing debt on completion and 70% received a means-tested bursary. Less than 31% held three or more A levels[7] and 29% completed an Access entry course. This presents a markedly different profile to the student cohort entering medicine.[8] On this basis we have used the concept of 'Ethical Education Placements' (EEPs) to distinguish them from 'electives', recognising that 'choice' always takes place within an environment of constraints. This also usefully distinguishes EEPs from forms of gap year 'voluntourism' facilitated through the growth of highly profitable companies as a component of tourism rather than education. The concept of 'voluntourism' is discussed in more detail in Chapter 5.

The second major ethical concern is with impacts in host (low resource) settings. Central to our discussion is a consideration of how sending institutions and students can avoid causing harm to host institutions and the communities they serve. In other words, we are concerned with the ethics and ethical practices of electives when there are power differentials between high and low resource settings. The aims of the book therefore are twofold; firstly, through our analysis of rich qualitative data generated with students, sending institutions and host institutions in Uganda and India, we provide new knowledge of the learning and impacts of international educational placements. Secondly, we present the Ethical Educational Placement Project (EEP) as a model embodying a set of guiding principles for ethical policy and practice in international educational placements across multiple disciplines. We now introduce the reader to the idea of the elective, its conceptualisation and the different forms they take before examining the EEP concept.

---

[7] A-levels are the qualification that most young people take at the age of 18 in the UK as the primary means of accessing university.

[8] For further discussion of the impact of social class on educational choices.

## INTERNATIONAL HEALTH ELECTIVES

Since the 1970s and 1980s in particular, international health electives have been a feature of undergraduate university medical education. Electives provide students with the opportunity to gain experience 'in different cultural and clinical climates and have the opportunity to explore parts of the world that interest them' (Dowell and Merrylees 2009: 122). There are different curricula elements to prepare students for electives, and various models exist which can have different impacts on student learning and host communities (Murdoch-Eaton and Green 2011). Electives can be a few weeks or a few months in duration and usually have a clinical focus, whether that is related to direct clinical practice or more towards data collection, audit or research which can feed into dissertation or publication writing. Some students engage in hands-on clinical practice during electives. There is growing pressure to regulate this in an increasingly risk aware (and potentially risk averse) environment with concerns about insurance, supervision, indemnity and liability. Placements for those students not allowed to engage in clinical practice are usually observational in nature. Aside from the clinical settings, more 'packaged' electives such as those offered by for-profit organisations may include either compulsory or optional cultural 'add-ons' or experiences which enable students to engage in learning foreign languages, crafts or tourist activities. Travel forms a key part of most electives and students often arrange personal holidays before, during or after their 'core' placement.

The potential gains of electives for students are well-documented (see Brookfield 1995; Elit et al. 2011; Murdoch-Eaton and Green 2011) and encompass in general terms, both professional and personal development and the acquisition of new knowledge in and of different contexts (Ackerman 2010). In more specific terms, these positive impacts for students are believed to include: the development of clinical skills in a new context; knowledge of and experience in different health systems; professional development; the development of generic skills, including organisational skills, communication, negotiation, self-evaluation, cultural competence, compassion towards patients, awareness of resource use, confidence, goal setting, widening students' perspectives, independence and personal growth; reflective questioning of both the challenges and assumptions of practices; greater understanding of different value systems; and 'social accountability' (Brookfield 1995; Elit et al. 2011) leading to a range of 'socially responsible' educational outcomes (Murdoch-Eaton and Green 2011).

However, throughout the book we question whether it is possible for students to unproblematically acquire such skills and attributes since merely participating in an elective does not necessarily guarantee compassion and competence, cultural or otherwise. Furthermore, a lack of understanding of the broader structural processes at play may preclude meaningful reflection (Hanson et al. 2011). There are concerns across a number of disciplines, including nursing, dentistry, veterinary and social work, that electives are a form of 'benevolent imperialism' (Razak 2002 cited in Huish 2012) contributing to Western students' assumptions of superiority (Elit et al. 2011). This in turn undermines the achievement of socially responsible outcomes. We discuss this in more detail below. In the following chapters, we also problematise the concepts 'cultural awareness' and 'cultural competence' and frame this discussion within the context of historical structural inequality between high resource and low resource settings (Hanson et al. 2011) and the differences in the positionalities[9] of students from high resource settings and students/health workers in low resource settings.

## THE ETHICAL EDUCATIONAL PLACEMENT (EEP) CONCEPT

There is a growing literature on the challenges of integrating ethically sound global health training into research and educational partnerships (see for example Dowell and Merrylees, 2009; Petrosoniak et al. 2010; Hanson et al. 2011; Huish 2012; Dasco et al. 2013). International medical electives are demand driven: some students have altruistic motivations and want to have the experience of serving in resource poor settings, while others are more career motivated and want to enhance their CVs (Huish 2012). On a global scale, medical schools and gap-year companies have responded to this increase in demand but ethical considerations have not kept pace, resulting in two broad challenges. First, in relation to the hubris[10] of Western

---

[9] The term 'positionality' is used in social science to refer to the 'adoption of a particular position in relation to others usually with reference to issues of culture, ethnicity, or gender' (https://en.oxforddictionaries.com/definition/positionality).

[10] Excessive pride or self-confidence (https://en.oxforddictionaries.com/definition/hubris).

(medical) students; and second, the creation and perpetuation of structural dependency for host countries and inequalities between sending and hosting countries (Huish 2012). Although the benefits of electives for students are widely recognised, the returns to students often outweighs the benefits to host organisations (Elit et al. 2011). It is becoming increasingly apparent that there are educational and moral reasons to develop more considered and ethical approaches to the design and operation of electives to avoid the pitfalls of medical or poverty tourism (Dowell and Merryless 2009) and minimise the potential harm caused to host communities (Petrosoniak et al. 2010).

Most research on the ethics of electives has focused on international placements in medical education with a primary focus on student experience and safety (Huish 2012). The British Medical Association (BMA 2009) guidelines on ethics in medical electives focus primarily on issues of competency arguing that students should always act within their competence even when dealing with emergencies. The guidelines also emphasise the importance of maintaining ethical standards required in home placements with an emphasis on honesty and integrity, dignity and respect, non-discrimination, prioritisation of patient needs, confidentiality and communication. The guidelines do recognise the importance of cultural openness and the potential burden on the host country but there is little specification of what this means and how it should be handled. The BMA is clear that medical students are not doctors, and that the main benefits for them are an increase in global health knowledge and understanding health service provision in another context: the acquisition of new clinical skills is not seen to be the goal. However, the development of clinical skills is often expressed as a motivation for students or as an intended outcome of electives (see for example Murdoch-Eaton and Green 2011).

It remains apparent then that there is uncertainty and a lack of clarity on behalf of students, sending and host organisations about how to ensure best practice on electives. Despite guidelines, while navigating different medical cultures, students often work out of and beyond their competencies (Elit et al. 2011). There is also concern that the presence of elective students can be a burden on systems already struggling to manage patients with limited staffing and scarce resources (Hanson et al. 2011; Huish 2012). In this way, electives may exploit low resource settings. Significantly, the important issues of whether electives can better meet the healthcare needs of host countries and their contribution to global health remains under-researched, and feature less in discussions of ethics.

Planning and preparation of the elective is important in order to avoid 'voluntourism' approaches as this will negatively impact on both the learning opportunities available and the host country. It is generally accepted that for electives to be ethical, there needs to be genuine partnerships between sending and host organisations, and the establishment of mutually agreed goals to ensure that host settings are not exploited (Murdoch-Eaton and Green 2011). Dasco et al. (2013) propose a 'host country first approach' which focuses on social justice, academic equity, exchange, transparency, cultural competence and the establishment of mutual defined goals. Huish (2012) calls for a restructuring of international health electives curricula to incorporate issues around social science and moral ethics pedagogy and clarify how 'global health inequity is ultimately a social constructed, anthropocentric phenomenon' (2012: 14). Hanson et al. (2011) further suggest that Western students and host institutions need to have or develop 'epistemic humility.'[11] We revisit these issues when we present the Ethical Educational Placement Project in Chapter 2. It is important that the curriculum, augmented by pre-departure training for those who do travel, prepares students to understand the context in which they will be placed (Murdoch-Eaton and Green 2011; Huish 2012). In other words, for educational placements to be ethical, students and sending organisations need to have a deep understanding of the environment and the application of concepts and values such as justice, power, fairness, cultural knowledge and self-awareness (Hanson et al. 2011). Further work with students on their return is critical to optimisation of learning. Mentorship is also an integral part of ethical placements and students need proper mentorship, informed and structured by ethical considerations (Ackerman 2010; Huish 2012). Finally, for educational placements to be ethically conducted and educationally efficacious for students, there is a need for explicit attention to their design, delivery and evaluation (Clampin 2008; Murdoch-Eaton and Green 2011).

## THE REMAINDER OF THE BOOK

Chapter 2: *The Ethical Educational Placement Project* describes the development, conceptualisation and operationalisation of the Ethical Educational Placement Project and identifies participating student cohorts and Higher

---

[11] Indicating an uncertainty about what you know, not assuming that what you know is more important than what others know.

Education Institutions (HEIs). We also summarise the evidence base for the presentation of a suggested 'model' for the development of EEPs.

Chapter 3: *Student Learning on Ethical Educational Placements* focuses on what students learn from educational placements in low resource settings. The term 'learning' is used quite fluidly to embrace wider experiential learning – what students often describe as 'life changing' or 'transformational impacts' and more specific curriculum or employment relevant skills.

Chapter 4: *Ethical Placements? Under What Conditions Can Educational Placements Support Sustainable Development?* focuses on the ethical aspects of the EEP concept to ask how and in what circumstances can hosting students from high resource settings be of benefit to low resource settings.

Chapter 5: *Managing Reciprocity: No Harm Approaches to International Educational Placements* draws together the research findings and reflects on what they contribute to the development of a more coherent body of knowledge about student mobility and especially student experiences in low resource settings. It ends with a summary of the key ingredients of Ethical Educational Placements.

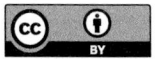

# CHAPTER 2

# The Ethical Educational Placement Project

## INTRODUCTION

In the introduction, we highlighted that international health electives have been a growing feature of medical education since the 1980s (Banerjee 2010) and that these are now viewed as important contributions to a diverse range of health-related undergraduate programmes. It is widely accepted that electives are beneficial to and popular with students (see, for example, Hastings et al. 2014), and that they have positive impacts on skills acquisition, personal and professional development, and knowledge of medicine and healthcare systems in different contexts. Electives are also considered to be important for students to learn about preventative health and social responsibility, so there are identified humanitarian as well as academic, professional and clinical benefits (Ackerman 2010). However, we emphasised that there are limited meaningful assessments of the outcomes gained on placements. Importantly, little attention has been paid to the ethical issues faced by students and, in particular, the impact of electives on host organisations, communities and countries.

## THE BACKGROUND

The development of the Ethical Educational Placement (EEP)project originated from the experiences of the Liverpool-Mulago Partnership (LMP). In 2010, LMP held a workshop in Liverpool inviting

© The Author(s) 2017      15
A. Ahmed et al., *The Ethics of Educational Healthcare Placements in Low and Middle Income Countries*, DOI 10.1007/978-3-319-48363-4_2

representatives of other UK Uganda health partnerships. This resulted in the setting up of the Ugandan Maternal and Newborn Hub (HUB)[1] whose role it was to support individual health partnerships through knowledge sharing and, where appropriate, volunteer mobility. One of the first actions we undertook was a HUB-wide benchmarking process to capture, as accurately as possible, facility-based data on admissions and services. This provided our first opportunity to trial student placements and we deployed 12 students from the University of Liverpool, placing them in pairs in HUB facilities and tasking them to work with local records managers to build capacity in records management and data collection. This provided the basis for our first HUB-wide benchmarking Report. Both Ackers and Ackers-Johnson accompanied the students on this ambitious project.[2]

At this time, and building on our successful model of professional volunteer deployment, we successfully applied for funding to set up the Sustainable Volunteering Project (SVP).[3] The SVP was a professional volunteering project funded by the Department for International Development (DfID) through the Tropical Health and Education Trust (THET). The SVP deployed 55 long-term Professional Volunteers[4] (PVs) from medical, nursing, midwifery, engineering and social science backgrounds to nine health facilities spread across Uganda over a three-year period between April 2012 and March 2015. Each PV engaged in knowledge exchange and capacity-building activities, such as classroom training sessions, workshops and on-the-job mentoring in order to share skills and make improvements to their personal practice and the Ugandan Public Healthcare System.

Throughout the SVP, PVs frequently reported instances of poor practice relating to the organisation and implementation of international – usually medical – student elective placements in their facilities.

---

[1] The Tropical Health and Education Trust provided financial support to establish the HUB.

[2] The results of this are reported in Ackers-Johnson (2010).

[3] For more detailed information on the SVP and the impact of professional voluntarism on LMICs, see Ackers and Ackers-Johnson (2016).

[4] We have used the term 'Professional Volunteer' to refer to qualified professionals deployed for periods of three months to over three years. We critique the use of the term 'volunteer' to accurately describe these roles in Ackers et al. (2016).

Students would often arrive seemingly unannounced at health facilities and engage in unsupervised, unstructured and often risky activities. Many were reported to be acting over and above their level of training and competency, potentially putting themselves and their patients at risk. Some students worked unpredictably, appearing only sporadically between various safari excursions and mountain treks, reinforcing the negative and often damaging 'voluntourism' stereotype. Others struggled to build relationships and integrate into the local facilities, leading to unproductive and disappointing placements. On many occasions, PVs found themselves supervising and supporting international students during their placements, despite them making financial payments to private and host organisations for such services. During the SVP, a number of students approached the LMP directly for assistance in organising medical elective placements in Uganda; many had discovered the LMP's activities online and wished to get involved in ongoing projects. The LMP assisted in organising the logistics of these placements, the majority of which were self-funded. PVs played a key role in assisting in the placement planning process and providing mentoring and supervision during the placements.

The impacts of the students' placements were monitored in terms of their effects on the PVs, the hosting facilities and their personal placement satisfaction and learning outcomes. The results were very positive; students benefitted greatly from having the PV to guide, supervise and educate them which improved learning outcomes. The PVs appreciated having the students working with them as they often offered fresh insights, inspiration and motivation. Any potential damaging effects on the hosting facilities were minimised; patients were put at less risk and the students conducted concrete, meaningful placements devised in conjunction with the LMP and the local facilities which were of mutual benefit to all parties. These overwhelmingly positive results formed the basis of the EEP; linking structured short-term student placements to long-term professional volunteer placements to design and implement sustainable interventions.

Despite the success of the SVP and the positive impacts of the PVs on the Ugandan Healthcare System, the project came to an end in March 2015 as continuation funding could not be secured. This is a problem associated with project funding which is often relatively short-term and unpredictable. However, through the student placements an opportunity to create a self-sustaining model which was not reliant on precarious funding streams was identified. The vast majority of international student elective placements are funded by the students themselves and are organised through private organisations such as 'Work the World'. As indicated in the introduction, very little research has been conducted into the impact of educational placements; including their ethics, learning outcomes, sustainability and value for money. This highlighted a gap in the international student placement market for supervised, risk assessed and effective educational placements which focused on mutual learning, safety, sustainability, ethics and positive local impact.

## THE CONCEPT

A concept paper was written by members of the SVP project management team based at the University of Salford (UK), in collaboration with colleagues at Mountains of the Moon University (MMU) in Uganda and trustees from a UK based charity, Knowledge for Change (K4C).[5] The objectives of the EEP concept were to establish, operationalise and develop ethical and sustainable undergraduate educational placements, capable of enhancing public health services in Uganda, whilst also providing optimal placement experiences and learning outcomes for British and Ugandan undergraduates and the professionals working with them.

Fort Portal was selected as the primary Ugandan placement site because of K4C's ongoing relationship with Kabarole Health District, Buhinga Regional Referral Hospital, Mountains of the Moon University and the University of Salford. This relationship had been formalised two years previously, with a Memorandum of Understanding in place outlining expectations, roles and responsibilities. Fort Portal was judged to be one of the safest places in Uganda to host student placements in terms of its location, road safety and the local environment. Additionally, there were relatively few international organisations working in Fort Portal, compared to places such as Gulu, Kisiizi and Kampala, which meant not only could our project (including PVs) have more of an impact on the local area but also any impacts on the students or local area would be more easily attributable.

---

[5] K4C is a registered charity (registered charity no. 1146911) in both the UK and Uganda, committed to stimulating improvements in well-being and livelihoods in Uganda by strengthening public services and systems through partnership and the mutual exchange of knowledge.

The first phase of the project aimed to build directly on relationships established and experienced gained during the SVP and focused on public health systems. This would include improving public access to health services, improving the quality of services and patient outcomes, improving referrals systems in order to reduce delays in accessing health services, and reducing patient congestion in referral hospitals. A comprehensive evaluation of the SVP had previously identified a number of key challenges facing the Ugandan Healthcare system, which included:

- Human resource management systems were characterised by high levels of absenteeism, 'moonlighting' and very low levels of employee motivation.
- Improvements in initial degree level education.
- Increased opportunities for, and equitable access to, relevant continuing professional development.
- Management of physical resources such as infrastructure, transport, drugs and other consumables.
- Empowerment of patients through improved information and communication systems.
- Improved evidence-based approaches based on evaluation, record-management and audit.
- Identification of tools to improve accountability and good governance.

To achieve the aforementioned objectives, the organisation of the EEPs was aligned with a holistic framework of priorities. The first priority was to enhance patient wellbeing through improvements in the referral systems. This would be achieved by targeting local facilities at key points in the public referral system which were not fully functional, but whose functionality could be restored with minimal resource intervention. The overall goal of this intervention was to reduce congestion in larger health facilities further down the referral pathway, such as the regional and national referral hospitals. The second priority was to support continuing professional development (CPD) for local staff and students; this would be achieved through the deployment of experienced professional PVs to provide and sustain CPD (known as Continuing Medical Education or CMEs in Uganda). PVs would contribute to initial education by co-teaching on local degree programmes to invest in the current workforce. This linked to the first priority of enhancing patient well-being through increasing referrals, as functioning facilities are essential to effective volunteer engagement and to ensure co-presence with local staff. The third priority was to support Higher Education systems in Uganda. The project would support a local partner, Mountains of the Moon University (MMU), in the delivery of undergraduate and graduate level education and the design and operationalisation of new degrees in Nursing and Midwifery to invest in the future workforce. Again, having functional facilities is critically important in enabling effective education and training, especially in placement settings. The locations highlighted in priority one would be carefully selected to ensure that they could act as effective placement training sites for MMU students.

The fourth priority was to provide structured educational placements with enhanced learning outcomes. The knowledge and experience gained during the SVP provided the basis for the operationalisation of a programme of student placements. These were to be structured and managed to minimise risk and enhance learning outcomes and were negotiated to ensure that they supported local services and objectives including: local health facilities, MMU education programmes and capacity-building in evaluation. The placements would be operated on a not-for-profit basis and would be jointly managed by UK and Ugandan institutions and partners with full co-ownership and co-stewardship in place. The fifth and final priority was to support evidence-based policy transfer; ensuring effective evaluation and dissemination to encourage similar initiatives in other areas of Uganda and elsewhere.

A funding application, along with the EEP concept paper, was submitted to Health Education England's 'Global Health Forerunner' fund, proposing the aforementioned EEP model for international educational placements for Nursing, Midwifery and Allied Health Professional students and funding was requested to pilot 40 such placements in Fort Portal, Uganda, over a 12-month period. Negotiations with HEE led to the inclusion of an additional 40 elective placements in India to be used as a comparison setting.[6] It was also decided that the placement opportunities should be opened up to Universities from across the North West of

---

[6] Although we supported the organisation and delivery of the India placements, these were included at the request of the funding body. K4C had no prior engagement or experience with projects in India. The placements were organised on an observation-only basis in a private not-for-profit facility. We extended our evaluation system to these placements to provide an element of comparison.

the UK and, on this basis, the funding was approved. The initial placement location selected for India was New Delhi, however risk assessments carried out during staff scoping visits judged this location to be too dangerous for students, in terms of both the city itself and the huge congested hospital facility. A smaller and safer city and hospital facility were selected; MS Ramaiah Hospital in Bengaluru. Bengaluru was identified as one of the safest and cleanest cities in India which made it more appropriate for hosting a large number of UK students. The placements were to be evaluated in terms of the students' learning outcomes and the impact of the placements on Uganda and India and their respective health systems. The end result was to devise a cost-effective model for student placements in low-income settings that could be up-scaled in Uganda and India, and potentially replicated elsewhere.

## PROJECT SETUP

The EEP project began on the 1 April 2015 with an official end date for the first phase of 31 March 2017. The initial stages of the project included various stakeholder meetings with partners in the UK, Uganda and India to discuss, negotiate and confirm the viability of the placement project and ensure the necessary levels of buy-in and support. As experienced during the SVP, strong and mutually beneficial relationships with clear reciprocal expectations are crucial when developing and sustaining projects of this nature in LMICs. The relatively hierarchical nature of organisations in Uganda and India increased the need for effective communication at multiple levels. In India, this included most importantly the director of M.S. Ramaiah Hospital and the principals of M.S. Ramaiah's Schools of Medicine and Nursing. In Uganda, where we had already established relationships, negotiations were made at health district level with the Kabarole District Health Secretary and District Health Officer. Negotiations were also made with the directors of the various health facilities and organisations which would be hosting the students. These included: Mountains of the Moon University, Buhinga Regional Referral Hospital, Mulago National Referral Hospital, Virika Hospital, Bukuuku Health Centre, Kibiito Health Centre, Kagote Health Centre, Kataraka Health Centre, Kyaninga Children's Development Centre, SOS Children's Village, Good Shepherd School, the Agency for Community Development and Welfare, the Youth and Women Empowerment Foundation and Baylor Uganda.

## RISK ASSESSMENT

Whilst stakeholder meetings and negotiations were taking place, comprehensive risk assessments were carried out at each of the proposed placement locations. These assessments updated and built upon a risk assessment of the SVP locations in Uganda completed by the Chief Risk Officer and Head of Global Health at the University Hospital of South Manchester in 2012,[7] highlighting and analysing risks to inform mitigation strategies for personal risks for the students and organisational risks for the University of Salford and K4C. The risk assessments for Uganda and India yielded relatively similar results, with road traffic accidents being identified as the greatest risk to the health and well-being of students and vicarious liability[8] being the greatest organisational risk. Other risks identified included assault and theft, illness resulting from unsafe food and drink, exposure to infection and tropical diseases, terrorism, civil unrest, the risk to students arising from unsafe or unsupervised clinical activities, getting lost in unfamiliar surroundings and excessive sun exposure.

The risk assessment was key to the design and implementation of the EEP, leading to the implementation of a variety of measures to mitigate the risks highlighted. For example, risk assessed accommodation was selected to host the students, safe and reliable transport was arranged for students between the airport, their accommodation and their placement locations. Also, rules regarding student travel outside of placement time were introduced to reduce the risk of road traffic accidents. To reduce the organisational risk of vicarious liability, policies were drawn up governing student placement activities and the required levels of supervision. The risk assessment advised that a single comprehensive insurance policy cover all the staff, PVs and students involved in the project to ensure an adequate level of cover for all parties and avoid them having to trawl through multiple different policies in the case of an emergency which may cause confusion and delays. Fortunately, the University of Salford's insurance

---

[7] The risk assessment is discussed in more detail in Ackers et al. (2016) and is available on the K4C website: www.knowledge4change.org.uk

[8] Vicarious liability refers to a situation where someone is held responsible for the actions or omissions of another person. In a workplace context, an employer can be liable for the acts or omissions of its employees, provided it can be shown that they took place in the course of their employment.

policy was judged to be suitable for this purpose and was able to provide the necessary cover.

Over the course of the EEP, there has been only one instance in which the insurance policy was required; this occurred when a student in India aggravated an existing back injury, possibly whilst driving on a bumpy road or carrying luggage up a flight of stairs to their accommodation. The insurance policy worked well; the student received the necessary treatment at a high-quality private hospital in Bengaluru before being returned to the UK with a medical escort. We had not been aware of the back injury prior to the placement commencing; this led to the implementation of a written medical questionnaire, given to students prior to their placements, requiring the disclosure of any physical or mental health conditions that they are aware of. It was made clear that failure to do this could cause serious individual problems, destabilise the whole placement group and potentially void the insurance policy putting the individual and organisation at risk.

Where a pre-existing medical condition was declared, advice was sought from both the insurers and the PVs on the ground in the placement location as to the suitability and viability of the placement. The opinion of the PV was particularly important as they had experience and knowledge of the local health system and would also often be the first port of call in any emergency situation. We took careful steps to support a number of students who disclosed health problems, for example autism and deep vein thrombosis, and the placements passed successfully. There was only one instance in which a student was refused a placement; this was due to a complex long standing heart condition which, although insurable, was judged by the PV to pose excessive risk as it could not have been treated locally should the condition have worsened during the student's placement. Naturally, the principle of equality of opportunity was always respected despite any disclosures and placements were only refused as a last resort. Both risk and insurance formed core elements of the student induction process which is explained in greater detail below.

## Student Recruitment and Selection

Once initial stakeholder meetings and negotiations had been completed, information on the project was circulated to the programme leaders for each discipline at each university; it was their responsibility to share this information with necessary staff and students within their respective institutions. Students were initially invited to attend an information day, during which they were given more general information about the project including what it would involve, our expectations, logistics and the timeframes of the placements. There was a great deal of interest and, almost immediately, large numbers of applications were received from students.

The application and selection process comprised three main stages; the first stage involved each student submitting a completed written application form consisting of three main sections, the first being basic personal information. The second section asked students to answer three questions in no more than 250 words each. The first question related to their reasons for applying for a placement, the second question asked what they hoped to achieve and experience during their placement, and the third question asked how they believed the placement would impact on their learning and future employability. The final section of the application form required students to select their preferred placement dates which varied from cohort to cohort. The candidates who submitted the highest quality application forms and suited the eligibility criteria relating to their university, study discipline and level of study were invited for interview. Achieving a representative sample of students from the multiple different institutions, disciplines and study levels was extremely challenging given that each group had conflicting 'mobility windows' (times in the year at which they could travel) and the need for the project to begin immediately and be completed within an 18-month period. Midwifery students in particular struggled to find time within their academic and UK placement timetables to be able to complete a four-week placement and some had to use some of their annual leave allowance. The need for flexibility increases further when placements are part of the curriculum and are assessed. Rather than sticking to rigid placement timings, the EEP placements offered flexibility throughout the year to try to accommodate as wide a group of students as possible.

Although the EEP evaluation strongly suggests that all students, at any stage in their degree programme, have benefitted hugely from their placement, the optimal placement timing was found to be towards the end of their penultimate year of study. These students tended to have a better attitude towards learning than less advanced students and were better able to share their learning and experience with peers upon their return to the UK (students completing placements at the end of their final year would tend to move straight into employment roles). These students were also better able to contribute to the low resource setting as a result of their higher level of academic knowledge and workplace experience. Many of the students were mature students who had previous experience and/or degrees; these students tended to show greater resilience and confidence and were able to contribute more to local facilities. Therefore, in terms of the selection process, students in their second year of study onwards (with the exception of Masters' level students) were preferred.

The interview processes consisted of both individual and group interviews which were moderated by members of the project management team. The main qualities sought during the interviews were communication skills, team working skills, leadership skills, resilience and motivation. Again, building on SVP experience, these skills were deemed to be the most important in ensuring that students were able to cope emotionally and work efficiently during their placements. As a final stage of selection, the relevant programme leaders and/or personal tutors for each student were contacted to ensure that the student was able to travel on the selected dates and that there were no circumstances unbeknown to the project management team that would prevent the student from undertaking a placement, or expose the student or project to unacceptable levels of risk. Such circumstances expressed during the project included potential exam resits, outstanding coursework submissions, poor academic performance, poor attendance and health issues which had not been disclosed by the students themselves. Not all of these circumstances led to placement offers being withdrawn; for instance, some coursework deadlines were extended to enable students to complete the placement.

Over 350 application forms were received from students over the course of the project, and over 200 students were interviewed. The selection process was far more competitive for certain disciplines than others depending on the number of applications received, the dates of travel and the number of placements available. The most competitive discipline was usually adult nursing; one particular round of selection saw over 40 applications for just four placements. Other courses, such as podiatry, received very few applications which meant the majority of applicants were successful. There were a number of other factors which affected the number of applications received, the main being the methods and timing of information dissemination about the project within each institution and discipline, and the course structures and mobility windows available.

## Student Induction

A formal induction process was held for successful applicants, and this began approximately ten weeks before their placement start date. The first stage of this process was the dissemination of a comprehensive 'Induction Pack', 'Local Guide', a short film and a local phrase book which contained detailed information about many aspects of the placements including the locations, logistics and travel arrangements, health and safety, emergency contact details, code of conduct and disciplinary procedures, insurance, leisure activities, finances, language, food and drink, dress and cultural sensitivity. Similar topics were covered again during a compulsory 'Induction Day' which was four hours in duration and run approximately six weeks before the placement start date. The Induction Day provided further information to the students and enabled them to ask any questions they had. Where possible, visiting colleagues from the LMIC hosting institutions were invited to provide input and advice. The induction session gave students the opportunity to meet the placement group with whom they would be placed prior to travelling. This was greatly appreciated by the students who often formed groups on social media to stay in touch, offer peer support and arrange weekend activities, as the following quote illustrates:

> It has been nice to have that support since the induction, [our group] have been talking for a few weeks now and we have a good grasp of each other's personalities. It's good that we are going out as a team now as opposed to getting there and having to become a team (Nurse, Uganda)[9]

Students were also provided with 'EEP Placement Agreements' (Appendix 1) to read, sign and return. These formally outlined our expectations of them whilst on placement, such as hours of work and conduct. A final induction and orientation session was held for the students once they arrived at their placement location which involved a tour of the accommodation; local area and health facilities; the provision of a mobile phone and local sim card for emergency usage; an introduction to their long-term volunteer supervisors and local staff in placement facilities; and further information about the placements and what to expect.

---

[9] Sample characteristics are provided in Table 2.1. Where appropriate we give the discipline and location of the respondents in brackets after the quote. Unless otherwise stated, these refer to the students.

## PLACEMENT COHORTS AND LOCATIONS

All cohorts of students were accompanied on their flights to Uganda or India by a member of the EEP team; this proved important especially when small problems arose such as delayed flights and lost baggage. If flights arrived in the late afternoon or evening, students were accommodated at a secure hostel near the airport and travelled to their placement location the following morning. A number of students were anxious about travelling at night, even when accompanied by members of staff. Students were always collected from and returned to the airport by a known and trusted driver.

Over the course of the project, 111 students completed four-week educational placements in Uganda ($n$ = 92) and India ($n$ = 19). The number of placements in India was reduced from the proposed 40–19 due to logistics and timeframes; only one cohort could be run per year (in November) to coincide with M.S. Ramaiah's 'International Student Winter School Programme'. The remainder of the placements allocated for India were instead run in Uganda. The sample included students from 11 different Higher Education Institutions; University of Salford ($n$ = 49), University of Central Lancashire ($n$ = 19), Liverpool John Moore's University ($n$ = 15), Edge Hill University ($n$ = 12), Liverpool Hope University ($n$ = 4), Lancaster University in partnership with Central Manchester Foundation Trust ($n$ = 4), University of Cambridge ($n$ = 2), University of Cumbria ($n$ = 2), University of Glasgow ($n$ = 2), Anglia Ruskin University ($n$ = 1) and Queen Mary's University ($n$ = 1).

The first three cohorts of students, 36 in total, completed four week educational placements in Uganda between June and September 2015. The fourth cohort of six students and the fifth cohort of 19 students completed placements in Uganda and India respectively in November 2015. Eight further cohorts, 50 students in total, completed placements in Uganda between March and October 2016. The students' disciplines and placement locations are provided in Table 2.1. With the exception of the Prosthetics, Orthotics and Biomedical Engineering students, all the placements in Uganda were run in Fort Portal. The placements for the Business /NHS Management Trainees were split between Kampala and Fort Portal. All the placements in India were run in Bengaluru and Kaiwara, as explained in more detail later.

The optimal size of each cohort was found to be between six and eight students. Larger groups can lead to financial economies of scale, however they tended to fracture internally resulting in tensions and the breakdown of relationships, which detracted from the overall placement experience.

**Table 2.1**    Students' disciplinary background, gender and placement locations

| | Placement location | | | |
| | Uganda | | India | |
| Discipline | Male | Female | Male | Female |
| --- | --- | --- | --- | --- |
| Adult Nursing | 5 | 17 | 2 | 13 |
| Midwifery | 0 | 14 | 0 | 2 |
| Children's & Young People's Nursing | 0 | 9 | 0 | 0 |
| Business/NHS Management Trainees | 2 | 6 | 0 | 0 |
| Mental Health Nursing | 0 | 5 | 0 | 2 |
| Social Work/Social Policy | 2 | 5 | 0 | 0 |
| Physiotherapy | 2 | 3 | 0 | 0 |
| Medicine | 0 | 4 | 0 | 0 |
| Prosthetics & Orthotics (in Kampala) | 1 | 3 | 0 | 0 |
| Integrated Practice (Nursing & Social Work) | 0 | 3 | 0 | 0 |
| Occupational Therapy | 0 | 3 | 0 | 0 |
| Paramedic | 0 | 3 | 0 | 0 |
| Podiatry | 0 | 2 | 0 | 0 |
| Bioscience/Human Biology | 1 | 1 | 0 | 0 |
| Biomedical Engineering (in Kampala) | 1 | 0 | 0 | 0 |
| **Sub totals** | 14 | 78 | 2 | 17 |
| **Totals** | 92 | | 19 | |

*Source*: Created by the authors.

Multi-disciplinary (mixed) placement groups were found to work well and provide exposure to new ideas and problem solving both within the UK team but also in their engagement with local health workers and systems. However, such groups demanded more complex project planning and tighter logistical management on the ground across multiple facilities. There was inevitably a greater strain on accommodation with larger groups and often students were required to share one bedroom between two, each bedroom containing two double beds. Only a small number of mature students expressed concerns about sharing bedrooms, however other shared facilities such as washrooms and kitchen areas did come under pressure, often becoming messy and attracting ants and mice despite the employment of daily cleaners. It is very important to ensure that accommodation is of adequate standard and that the students are comfortable, otherwise it can lead to disputes within the group and can have a strong effect on students' wellbeing and placement experience.

## PLACEMENT STRUCTURE AND ACTIVITIES IN UGANDA: THE ROLE OF THE PROFESSIONAL VOLUNTEER

As noted above, all students were accompanied on their journeys to both Uganda and India. The Ugandan placements are also supported by the services of a full-time Ugandan Placement Manager who is on site at all times to support the students and the various K4C projects. In addition to regular visits by the UK team and the presence of a local placement manager, Professional Volunteers (PVs) play an important, complex and multifaceted role in the design and structure of placement activities in Uganda. First, they form a crucial link between the students, project managers and the hosting facilities and institutions, and are responsible for students' safety and learning whilst on placement. They were able to supervise students during their placements providing on-the-job training, debriefing and support their wellbeing. Although logistically they cannot be co-present with each student at every point in time, they are readily available. Regular (daily and weekly) debriefings take place with the Placement Manager, the PVs and the students. This is particularly important in cases where students encountered patient deaths or 'near misses'. Students based on the neonatal units all witnessed neonatal deaths; in two cohorts, this happened on their first day. Of course, such deaths are traumatic in themselves and the way of dealing with dead neonates in Uganda shocked students; there were clear cultural differences regarding the care of the newborn and the contact between the mother and her dead baby. Time was spent during induction sessions discussing this in order to prepare students, but the fact remains that this will happen and students will find it stressful at first, as the quote below illustrates:

> It was very hard to deal with, even though we were told what it would be like and to expect to see death. I don't really think we could be more prepared for it because even if you told somebody all about it, if it actually happens to you it's different. (Nurse, Uganda)

All students have coped well in these circumstances during their EEP placements as a result of the high level of support the model provides. It is important to add that the students also provided strong support for the PV in similar circumstances. Indeed it is clear that the presence of UK students contributed significantly to the learning, experience and support available to professional volunteers. For example, midwifery students working alongside PVs often assisted with complex deliveries and particularly with neonatal care and resuscitation (areas where skills are often found lacking in Uganda). The PVs have really enjoyed mentoring the students, gaining motivation from this experience in what are often quite difficult environments. Students also provide strong social support for them and the project as a whole which contributes in important ways to the overall (integrated) sustainability of the EEP model as the quote from a PV suggests:

> I've felt much less isolated over the last few weeks and having the students here has really helped with that. (Professional Volunteer, Uganda)

The second benefit of having PVs on the ground derives from the relative longevity of their placements which enables them to build and maintain strong relationships with local stakeholders such as the district health officers, facility in-charges and local staff. This not only leads to the mutual development of new and exciting project ideas with Ugandan stakeholders, but also expedites the students' transition into local organisations, health facilities and staff groups enabling them to begin their placements immediately on arrival in Uganda. This also avoids the problem observed during the SVP relating to local staff often being suspicious of – and occasionally unwilling to work with – unfamiliar foreign staff and students. Third, the PVs played an 'anchoring' function to sustain project activities in between cohorts of students, allowing one cohort to easily and effectively continue the work of their predecessors, thus maintaining momentum and improving the efficiency of development activity. Fourth, the PVs provided training to local staff and students within health facilities and by teaching on Mountains of the Moon University's nursing and midwifery degree programmes. This marked a positive ethical and sustainable step towards ensuring mutual benefit to both Uganda and the UK. Finally, the PVs played a useful role in project evaluation; providing feedback about the successes and challenges face by the students and the impact the project was having on the local health systems.

The EEP directly funded a PV midwife to supervise the first three cohorts of students travelling to Uganda in the summer of 2015. When the midwife completed her placement, an obstetrician took her place and remained in post for 12 months until the end of the EEP. Obstetric/midwifery focused PVs were recruited since the majority of care in Uganda, particularly in smaller rural health centre 4s, is maternity focused, and other ongoing K4C projects were predominantly focused on maternal and new-born health. Given that students were not continuously deployed on the ground in Uganda, it meant that PVs had the capacity to assist with these other K4C projects, boosting the development impact of the charity. Fortunately, K4C had other PVs based in Uganda but primarily working on different projects. These PVs included two biomedical engineers based in Kampala. All of these PVs were willing and able to assist in supervising the students whenever necessary. This was particularly helpful when the group of prosthetics and orthotics students travelled out to Uganda. The active engagement of our sister bio-medical engineering project (see www.knowledge4change.org.uk) provided excellent opportunities for prosthetics and orthotics students to spend time in Kampala under the direct supervision of our PV in the large prosthetics and orthotics departments in Mulago Hospital and Kyambogo University. This demonstrates the benefits of having a number of diverse ongoing projects and a wide-ranging network of knowledge and relationships within the host country.

## LOCAL SUPERVISION

In practice, it is impossible in the Ugandan public heath setting to guarantee one-to-one supervision in all placement locations given the turnover of staff, shift patterns, absenteeism and also cultural attitudes towards the supervision of students.[10] We tried to work towards this over the course of the EEP through close engagement with local staff and facility management but by the end of the project it was still occasionally lacking. This is partly the reason why students were placed in pairs, wherever possible, and were required to report any incidences of lone working to the placement manager or PV as a matter of urgency. The level of local supervision received by students was monitored through the weekly reporting process, which required students to state how often (never, rarely, sometimes, usually or always) they had been

[10] Ugandan students rarely receive active supervision whilst on their placements.

working alongside Ugandan colleagues and whether they had any concerns about this. The most common responses for the first three cohorts of students in 2015 were 'rarely' and 'sometimes'. By the end of the project, this had improved to 'usually' with many students selecting 'always'. As a project, we successfully applied for a significant number of Commonwealth Professional Fellowships which enabled us to bring Ugandan colleagues working in these facilities over to the UK for periods of between one and six months. This has played a very valuable role in augmenting relationships[11] and exposing them to the environment in UK universities and hospitals. The Fellows continue to play a very valuable role in supporting student information days, awareness raising and induction processes.

In the evaluation, no students reported any concerns about the level of supervision they received from local staff since many received sufficient supervision from a PV. Students believed they could access supervision quickly should it be required as the following excerpt suggests:

> Obviously being a student and being unsupervised isn't ideal however if I ever had any questions or needed support I could always call [the PV] and she would inform me about what to do or come over if it was an emergency. (Child Nursing Student, Uganda)

In most situations, particularly during placement in the smaller health centres and community based organisations, students have worked alongside excellent local staff and other students in mutual learning contexts. Given the breadth of disciplinary backgrounds this has been a learning curve for the placement managers who are now in a better position to select placements and also anticipate situations where students may experience staff shortages and potential lone working. Responding to these situations has proved beneficial both to the students but also to local health systems enabling us to leverage improvements in staffing, in attitudes towards student supervision and staff behaviour. By emphasising the necessity of supervision during placements for the UK students we are pushing ahead a model of good

---

[11] We have received three Fellowships to support Ugandan midwives in one of our smaller EEP training sites.

practice for Ugandan students. Co-locating the students in training sites[12] is making this possible and efficient.

## FLEXIBILITY VERSUS STRUCTURE

The educational placements in Uganda offered considerable flexibility to students based on their study discipline and personal areas of interest. Following the induction session, each student was given the opportunity to describe their personal interests and the ideal type of placement they were hoping to undertake and the types of facility they would prefer to be based in. Although it was made clear that not all requests could be fulfilled and that all placements would be negotiated with the various stakeholders involved in the project, the students' preferences were taken into consideration during the placement planning process. The main factors influencing the students' placement activity were the needs of the health system requested by local stakeholders, informed by PV opinions and verified by K4C and University of Salford management to ensure activities rested within the longer term organisational objectives. Given the iterative nature of the project, we were able to make a number of changes over the lifetime of the project to ensure that the placements were optimised to best achieve our objectives.

There was a careful balance to be achieved between autonomy and structure, and the level of flexibility to allow the students within their placement schedules was often difficult to gauge. Nursing and midwifery students tended to expect higher levels of structure, support and supervision in line with their experience of placements in the UK. This contrasted with, for example, the NHS graduate management trainees who requested a higher degree of autonomy and medical students who expected – and often actively sought – more intense autonomous clinical exposure rather than wider systems-focused placements. Often students expressed a desire to be placed in many varying locations in order to gain as wide an experience as possible, but this caused a number of problems. First, it

[12] The concept of 'training sites' has come from the EEP. It has included the improvement of infrastructure and equipment in the health centres nominated so that students can be placed in contexts where there is at least basic functionality and, where possible, examples of and opportunities for good practice. In the process systems and services are also being improved for patients.

made it difficult for them to integrate into the local health teams and build up strong relationships and the level of trust required for efficient co-working. One local physiotherapist explained how they were able and willing to supervise two students coming for multiple consecutive days; however, when three or four students were coming on different days, they failed to build relationships and it took much more time and effort having to explain the same things repeatedly. In moving around frequently, students were perceived as 'voluntourists' rather than colleagues by local staff which made them more suspicious of new students and therefore less likely to engage.

A second problem caused by placing students in a variety of settings was the additional burden placed on the UK and Ugandan project management team. Communication became more difficult as did organising the resulting more complicated placement schedules, supervision and daily transport plans. Third, a number of students reported feeling disappointed that they had not achieved as much as they had hoped as a result of moving around too frequently and therefore not having sufficient opportunities to engage in useful, tangible and impactful projects. Finally, it was observed that giving students a certain level of timetabling structure meant they were better able to maintain a positive routine; students who moved placement locations on a regular basis often reported greater confusion and stress which negatively impacted on their wellbeing. Additionally, some of the student requests (to spend time in local schools for example) had tenuous links to their study disciplines. However, although the learning from such placements would not be as directly relevant to the students' courses, it was acknowledged that they could help improve the student's knowledge and experience of health, education and social systems in LMICs. A decision was made to allow students to have half a day on Fridays away from their formal placements to engage in such 'side placement' activities, providing they were beneficial for the students' learning and experience and did not lead to additional risks or expense.

## PLACEMENT TIMETABLING

As emphasised in their 'EEP Placement Agreement', students are required to complete a normal working week of 36 hours. Most student placements begin at 09.00 and end at 17.00; however some also began at 08.00 and ended at 16.00 to fit with the timings of the PV, local doctors' ward rounds or NGO community visits. The students were allowed 45 minutes for lunch each day. The importance of beginning and ending placements promptly was emphasised to the students as this served as a form of role modelling for local staff and students. Students were only allowed to complete placements at night if it was in their personal interest and adequate supervision and transport arrangements could be provided to minimise risk. The main risks of working at night, as highlighted by the risk assessment, include transportation to and from placement when it is dark and the increased aforementioned risks associated with students being left to work alone and without adequate supervision.

At the beginning of the project, students would be on placement for five full days per week. Report writing for the purposes of the project evaluation, group meetings and debriefing were conducted in the evenings and weekends. However, many students reported that they did not feel they had sufficient time to debrief and write their reports, particularly as they were spending relatively long hours on placement compared to the UK. In addition, they indicated that the placements were often more difficult and/or stressful as a result of increased numbers of traumatic experiences, more demanding working conditions and a more debilitating climate. Also, students often engaged in personal leisure activities or relaxation during evenings and weekends which put pressure on the free time they had. It was therefore decided that each Friday would be split, with the morning dedicated to the 'side placements' and the afternoon involving a team meeting between project managers, PVs and students, a reflection and debriefing session and time for report writing.

## STUDENT PLACEMENT ACTIVITIES

The majority of nursing and midwifery students competed hospital and health centre based placements. These included observational elements on the wards and theatres, along with hands-on clinical training under the supervision of the local staff and PVs across multiple facilities. Students were not permitted to work on their own without local or PV guidance for a number of reasons: this could potentially put them and the project at risk of litigation following medical malpractice as noted within the risk assessment; it does not foster efficient and mutual learning between the students and LMIC partners; and it detracts from the relationship building and team working. Students were generally placed in pairs as this reduced the risk of lone working, improved integration and simplified arrangements for supervision and transport. One Ugandan midwife reported how larger groups of students often found it more difficult to integrate into the local workforce as students tended to 'stick together' as a group. This midwife also explained how larger groups tended to be a *greater burden on both local staff and PVs in terms of their management and supervision* and could *occasionally intimidate local staff and patients who were not comfortable in dealing with large groups (of foreign students)*.

Initially the physiotherapy, occupational therapy and podiatry students also began placements in the hospital facilities. However, these were not successful for a number of reasons, the main one being that these professions were not well recognised in Uganda and therefore the students had little or no support from local staff. Also, staff working in the public sector, particularly in these less recognised areas, are often poorly paid, poorly managed and as a result poorly motivated and frequently absent. This meant the students – particularly the physiotherapy and occupational therapy students – were sometimes left unsupervised and finished their placements early each day. The gaps in the Ugandan health service left by these poor or non-existent services were often filled by the non-governmental organisation (NGO) sector funded and/or wholly run by international individuals and organisations. Using existing relationships and networks, we were able to locate and approach a number of these organisations and successfully negotiate the possibility of them hosting students. 'Kyaninga Children's Development Centre',[13] for example, proved to be an extremely successful placement location for physiotherapy and occupational therapy students. Similarly, the 'Youth and Women's Empowerment Foundation (YAWE)' NGO was able to provide effective placements for Nursing, Integrated Practice and Social Work students.

Other organisations hosting students on non-health focused placements included the Fort Portal Juvenile Centre, Fort Portal Open Prison, Kyaka II Refugee Settlement, Kyambogo University and Mountains of the Moon University (MMU). These organisations were particularly beneficial in hosting Social Work and Business students. A number of students from various disciplinary backgrounds (including health) ran teaching sessions for MMU students. These teaching sessions

---

[13] Kyaninga Children's Development Centre (www.kyaningacdc.org) is an NGO in Fort Portal which supports children with physical and mental disabilities such as cerebral palsy, cerebral malaria and brain injuries. They hosted six physiotherapy and occupational therapy students over the course of the EEP.

were negotiated and arranged by the UK students in partnership with MMU staff to ensure the content was relevant for the Ugandan students and could be taught to an acceptable standard. The sessions included (amongst others) lectures run by Social Work students on the potentially harmful effects of drugs and alcohol, workshops run by Midwifery students on safe childbirth, lectures run by Nursing students on infection prevention and control and lectures by NHS management trainees on the principles of management.

## PLACEMENT STRUCTURE AND ACTIVITIES IN INDIA

The placements in India were established and managed quite differently to those in Uganda, mainly due to the nature and history of the partnership. The partnership with M.S. Ramaiah Hospital was formed solely for placement purposes, rather than being an ongoing partnership focused on capacity building, health system development and sustainability. This meant that there were no existing networks, relationships, experience or knowledge to build upon. There were also no PVs on the ground to support the project's development or the students on their placements. The India placements offered more a more formal and rigid structure and far less flexibility for the students since the placement timetable, accommodation and transportation were all prearranged by M.S. Ramaiah Hospital with relatively little input from the UK project management team. In effect the placements were organised as a 'package' put together by the India leads and charged to the UK project.[14]

During the in-country induction, each UK student was paired up with an Indian 'buddy' whose role was to provide support and guidance during placements. The buddy system worked very well in most instances. All the buddies were studying similar courses to the UK students at M.S. Ramaiah Nursing School, and this enabled them to exchange knowledge and experience; they were particularly instrumental in overcoming language barriers and would translate conversations between doctors, nurses and patients. The UK students and their buddies often formed friendships, which gave them increased insights into each other's lifestyles and

---

[14] The package provided by M.S. Ramaiah was priced at £850 per student to include in-country accommodation, transport, supervision and food.

cultures. Socially, the buddies played a useful role in showing the students around the local area and advising them where to buy food and clothes.

The first two weeks of the placements were spent in M.S. Ramaiah Hospital, a large non-profit private hospital, where students observed on wards and in operating theatres alongside their buddies. Throughout the placements, the students were wholly supervised by local medical and nursing staff. Students were rotated through many varying hospital departments, offering wide ranging of clinical exposures. Students followed a prescheduled timetable whilst placed in the hospital, spending each morning in one location and rotating to a different location in the afternoon. Students were collected from their accommodation by bus at 08.15 each morning to begin their placements at 09.00. They were allowed 45 minutes for lunch then finished at 16.30 when they were returned to their accommodation. All the placements in India were observational only and the students were not permitted to engage in any hands-on care of patients. There were two main reasons for this; first, as the hospital environments were less familiar we could not guarantee a sufficient level of supervision for the students and therefore needed to avoid the risks related to lone-working. Second, the regulatory environment in India tends to be stricter than in Uganda. Both project management and Indian colleagues were keen to minimise the risk of litigation against the students arising from medical negligence or malpractice. This was made clear to the students during the induction process. However, the vast majority students expressed a strong desire in their feedback for hands-on clinical placements, stating its anticipated benefits for their own learning and their sense of efficacy and desire to 'make a difference' as the following quote illustrates:

> I just feel I could have contributed so much more if we were allowed [to engage in hands-on practice], it felt awkward just standing and watching when we could have been helping at least with basic, routine care like wound dressings and changing beds which we do all the time in the UK. (Adult Nursing student)

The second two weeks were spent attending the Gokula Education Foundation 'Winter School'. This was a formal residential school which took place in a rural town called Kaiwara. The 19 UK students were split into groups of four or five, within which they worked alongside a large number of medical students from M.S. Ramaiah's School of Medicine to conduct a wide range of projects designed to benefit the local community. Such projects included designing hand hygiene protocols and conducting training in infection prevention and control; devising plays and fun activities to deliver healthcare messages to small surrounding villages and schools; assisting local clinicians with patient assessment and treatment during health camps and assessing safe water collection and storage protocols. All the students appreciated being able to experience both placement locations and being able to compare and contrast the urban and rural settings. Each location offered differing placement activities, health facilities, cultures, environments, accommodation, placement groups and patient demographics. As with the placement in Bengaluru, all the accommodation, transport arrangements and placement activities were organised by M.S. Ramaiah through their Gokula Education Foundation.

## LEISURE AND FREE TIME

It was made clear to all students in both Uganda and India that the evenings and weekends could be used for their personal leisure and free time. The activities that the students completed during these times depended on their location, personal preferences and finances. In Uganda, the majority of students completed tourist activities such as safari trips, mountain hiking, touring crater lakes and visited a variety of sights and attractions. In India, the students went on an organised visit to a temple at Mysore, attended a traditional Indian wedding and visited local tourist attractions within Bengaluru. The students were allowed to take part in any activity provided it was covered by the insurance policy, was not judged to put them at risk and did not negatively affect their formal placements. Completing such leisure and tourist activities was found to be greatly beneficial to the students as it allowed them to relax, experience more of the culture and environment within the LMIC and generally improved their happiness and wellbeing. The only instances in which the project managers were required to intervene concerned students consuming excessive amounts of alcohol whilst socialising in bars and clubs in the local towns. On two occasions, students were warned that their behaviour put them at personal risk and that continuing to engage in such behaviour might lead to disciplinary action. As a result, an additional clause was added to the student placement agreement regarding the consumption of excessive amounts of alcohol and the potential risks and consequences.

Some students wanted to prolong the duration of their placements to allow for personal holiday time and this was permitted and flights were arranged accordingly. However, the students were required to pay any additional airfare and had to agree that any extra time spent in the placement country before or after their official placement was undertaken completely at their own risk and expense since the project would take no responsibility for them and they would not be covered by the University's insurance policy.

## PLACEMENT COSTS AND STUDENT CONTRIBUTIONS

The first five cohorts of students who completed their placements in Uganda and India over the course of 2015, with the exception of the self-funded students, received full funding. This covered the cost of flights, accommodation (including free Wi-Fi), visas, 'in country' airport transfers, placement transport, insurance, supervision and pastoral support, an emergency mobile phone with a local sim-card and a small amount of airtime and, in the Ugandan placements, a direct investment of £150 per student into the local host health facility. The only costs that these students faced personally were for vaccinations, antimalarial prophylaxis, UK airport transfers, food, drink, tourism and leisure activities. Only one student out of 52 in this group reported experiencing difficulties in raising sufficient funding to be able to complete a placement, although this was mainly as a result of family circumstances and them having to support a dependent family member using the income from their part-time job.

A decision was made in January 2016 to ask students to contribute £395 towards the cost of their placements. This decision was made following student feedback which indicated that the students themselves thought they should be required to contribute something towards the placement costs. The figure of £395 was determined by the students as they deemed this amount to be affordable and fair given the experience they were having and the relatively small costs they were incurring. Of course, the introduction of a student contribution improved the project's cost efficiency and meant placement opportunities could be offered to a greater number of students. It was also felt that asking the students to make a relatively small contribution would dissuade those students who were more interested in exploiting the attractive offer of a 'free' international trip without actually being committed to the objectives of the project. A number of complaints were received – from both a local host organisation and fellow UK students – about some students (who did not make a contribution towards the cost of their placement) who did not seem to care much about their placements and instead were more interested in taking photos with children for their social media pages or engaging in tourist activities. It was found that students who did make a contribution towards the cost of their placement demonstrated higher levels of interest, motivation and engagement with the project which led to improved outcomes both in terms of students' learning and also the impact they had on the hosting facilities.

Students in the nursing, midwifery and allied health professions were generally less able than medical students to draw on personal and family resources to fund electives; they were a more diverse group and many had families and undertook paid work to support their education. A small but significant number of these students could not have engaged in the placement if they had to contribute large amounts, although even these students said they would be able to fund £395 if they had around six months' notice and/or support with fund raising and applying for travel bursaries.

In total, 86 of the 111 students had their placements funded by Health Education England; of these 52 were fully funded and 34 made a contribution of £395 to K4C. The remaining 25 students completed the placements on a self-funded basis at a cost of £1495; however, 13 of these received bursaries of £1000 from the aforementioned contributions received by K4C, meaning they each contributed only £495. A large number of the self-funded students and the students who made a contribution are known to have received bursaries or travel grants from external sources, such as University student support services, to fund all or the majority of the cost of their placements. The figure of £1495 has been assessed to cover the full cost of each student placement in both Uganda and India based on a group of eight students travelling on four-week placements every month (not including the cost of UK project management time). Larger group sizes can achieve cost savings as a result of economies of scale in relation to student induction, airport transfers, in-country transport and accommodation (plus PV supervision in Uganda). However, the main cost of each placement is the flight cost which remains fixed between £450 and £650, becoming higher at peak times in the year (Fig. 2.1).

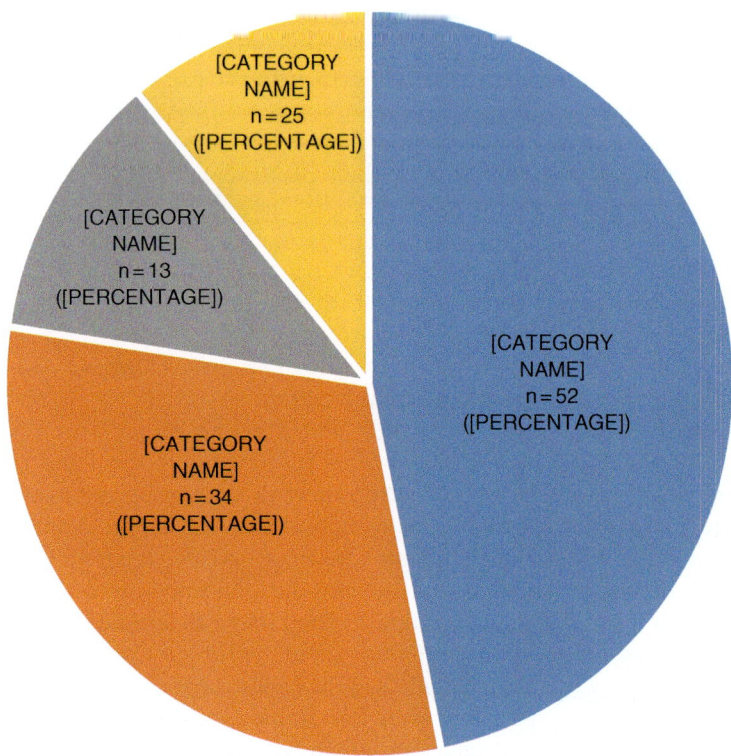

**Fig. 2.1**   Placement funding. *Source*: Created by the authors

## Project Evaluation

The fact that both the educational placements project and the wider health systems intervention in Uganda is based in an established research group (Knowledge and Place) at Salford University has supported high-level evaluation. The evaluation has taken a complex multi-method approach combining qualitative and quantitative methods. All of the data collected has been anonymised, coded and analysed using Nvivo10 software. A grounded approach was followed in generating a node framework, into which all qualitative data was imported and coded. The main sources of data collected during the EEP evaluation are summarised below:

- Weekly reports during placements.
- Comprehensive end of placement reports by all students.
- Pre-, mid- and post-placement interviews with all students.
- Post-placement survey sent out to all students.
- Interviews with UK HEI programme leaders.
- Interviews with Professional Volunteers (Uganda only).
- Interviews with staff in hosting LMIC facilities.
- Reports from staff in hosting LMIC facilities.
- Observations by UK and LMIC project management, evaluation staff and post-doctoral researchers.
- Transcribed focus groups, meetings and workshops with students, LMIC hosts, PVs and project management.
- Email communications between project management and PVs, students and hosting LMIC staff.

The pre-placement interviews aimed to assess how the students thought they would benefit from the placements and how these expectations related to their programme of study. They also focused on the financial implications of the placements and identified any areas where students may require additional support. The mid-placement interviews addressed practical issues such as placement logistics, supervision and student wellbeing; this informed the evaluation of the difficulties faced by students whilst on placement and the nature of pastoral care required to remedy any concerns. As the mid-placement interviews were carried out after just two weeks of the students being on placement, they did not focus so closely on learning outcomes or the impact the students perceived they were having on the LMIC. The post-placement interviews were carried out roughly a month after the students had returned to the UK from their placement. A month was found to be an appropriate delay before conducting the post-placement interviews as it gave the students the opportunity to settle back into regular life and reflect more clearly on their placements. Before, during and immediately after placements, students were sometimes overly focused on the short-term problems and stresses experienced over what was often a highly emotional four to six-week period for them, such as group dynamics, traumatic experiences and fatigue. Many students explained how their thoughts and feelings about their placements had changed hugely once they had had time to think and reflect properly, usually becoming more positive and continuing to do so the longer the time that elapsed after the placement.[15]

The weekly reports included questions about the students' general wellbeing, their roles and activities completed during the week, their learning and personal development, the extent to which they had been working under supervision and alongside UK and LMIC colleagues and any issues of concern they might wish to raise. The purpose of the weekly reports was two-fold; they informed the overall project evaluation and also provided an opportunity for students to raise any concerns which then enabled project management to take immediate action or make changes to placements. Many students used the written reports as useful form of reflection on the challenges they had faced during the preceding week and the actions they planned to take the following week to prepare for, avoid or overcome them. Similarly, the comprehensive end of placement student reports prompted the students to think back over their placement as a whole to summarise successes, achievements and challenges, and to provide productive feedback to inform necessary changes and improvements to the EEP.

The post-placement survey was designed using Survey Monkey and was disseminated to students over WhatsApp by means of a web link (Appendix 2). The survey was relatively short, comprised of only seven questions which aimed to collect quantitative data on the impact that the placements had on the students' learning, their future career and employability and on the LMIC. The survey also asked the students to rate their overall placement experience. Sixty-five responses were received in total when the survey was circulated in October 2016, which represented a response rate of 59% of the 111 students that completed placements.

Interviews were also conducted at regular intervals throughout the duration of the project with PVs and local hosting LMIC stakeholders. The main focus of these interviews was to establish the impact the student placements were having on the hosting LMIC and their constituent facilities, staff, health workers and patients. Interviewees were asked about both personal and professional impacts, as well as the impact they perceived the EEP to be having on their organisations and the health system

---

[15] Further research on the long-term impacts of midwifery placements is currently underway as part of Natalie Tate's doctorate; this will involve repeated interviews at six and twelve months post-return.

in general. The impact on the PV in terms of their learning, professional development and the impact their placement might have on the UK NHS was also evaluated (see Ackers and Ackers-Johnson 2016).

## SUMMARY

This chapter has described in some detail the operationalisation of the undergraduate educational placements that we have been involved with. The EEP model has evolved over time in an evidence-based fashion building on the experience of the Sustainable Volunteering Project and our experience then of managing a placement whilst also observing students on placement from other institutions across the world and the UK. We have included in this discussion the organisation of placements in India specifically requested by Health Education England. Having outlined the organisation of these placements and students' response to this, the following chapters move on to consider the outcomes and impacts associated with these kinds of placement.

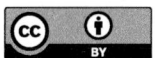

# CHAPTER 3

# Student Learning on Ethical Educational Placements

I grew in confidence and became a level headed professional, not just an awkward student. (Nurse, Uganda)

## TRANSFORMATIONAL LEARNING

As with the findings from our study of Professional Voluntarism,[1] it is difficult to isolate the different elements of learning experienced through placements since personal and professional skills overlap and some aspects of learning are almost intangible, particularly those transformational elements which characterise most students' accounts. The following two responses illustrate the transformational impacts as perceived by the students on placement:

I just feel like it's helped me change my outlook and personality. (Midwife, Uganda)

During my time there I went through a wave of different emotions from anger, frustration, passion, amazement and joy to name just a few...After returning home and having more time to reflect I believe that the experience had changed me on a level I wasn't expecting. (Nurse, India)

Fee and Gray capture the gains in capabilities and the value of skills gained in low resource settings to contemporary workplaces. They conclude that

---

[1] See Chapter 3 in Ackers and Ackers-Johnson (2016).

© The Author(s) 2017
A. Ahmed et al., *The Ethics of Educational Healthcare Placements in Low and Middle Income Countries*, DOI 10.1007/978-3-319-48363-4_3

such skills are not easily codified and taught: they are distinctively generic, rather than technical; tacit rather than explicit; higher order rather than basic; portable rather than profession or situation-bound and 'soft' (interpersonal) rather than 'hard' (technical):

> Notably, expatriates experienced learning outcomes that were more frequently transformational, involving fundamental changes to their values, perspectives or assumptions. (2013: 196)

There is strong evidence to suggest that stays in low resource settings create opportunities for accelerated and complex learning and that the outcomes of these are precisely the kinds of competences needed to drive innovation and efficiency in an increasingly resource-constrained NHS (Norton and Marks-Moran 2014). The potential gains of international elective placements for students are well-documented (see Brookfield 1995; Elit et al. 2011; Murdoch-Eaton and Green 2011) and encompass in general terms, both professional and personal development and the acquisition of new knowledge in and of different contexts (Ackerman 2010). In more specific terms, these positive impacts for students are believed to include: the development of clinical skills in a new context; knowledge of and experience in different health systems; professional development; the development of generic skills, including organisational skills, communication, negotiation, self-evaluation, cultural competence (Jeffrey et al. 2011), compassion towards patients, awareness of resource use, confidence, goal setting, widening students' perspectives, independence, and personal growth; reflective questioning of both the challenges and assumptions of practices; greater understanding of different value systems; and 'social accountability' (Brookfield 1995; Elit et al. 2011) leading to a range of 'socially responsible' educational outcomes (Murdoch-Eaton and Green 2011). Figure 3.1 summarises the findings of existing research on learning outcomes associated with international placements in low resource settings.

These domains map directly onto the UK's NHS Knowledge and Skills framework or 'KSF'.[2] The KSF is focused on staff development and appraisal and designed, 'to make it easier for staff to identify the core skills that they need to do their job and their development needs'. As such it is a

---

[2] http://www.nhsemployers.org/SimplifiedKSF

1. **Knowledge and Skills**
1.2 **Clinical (Academic) Knowledge**
   Substantive knowledge of contexts and health systems
   Resource awareness, management and efficiency
   Knowledge of research, evaluation and audit methods
2.2 **Clinical and Technical Skills**
   Exposure to a high volume of (usual) clinical cases and new (unusual) cases
   Generic, soft, interpersonal skills
   Organisational and administrative skills
2. **Values**
2.1 **Personal**
   Compassion/care
2.2 **Social**
   Ethics, morality, social responsibility, social accountability; global citizenship
   Equality and diversity
   Cultural competence
3. **Service improvement and Leadership**
   Problem solving, innovation and project management
   Team working including multi professional working
4. **Communication** (links to cultural competence and leadership)
   Teaching /presentational skills
   Negotiation
   Language skills
5. **Personal Growth and Professional Development**
   Confidence
   Goal setting
   Independence
   Self-evaluation and reflective questioning

**Fig. 3.1** Summary of learning outcomes. *Source*: This summary is drawn from the authors cited above complemented by Dowell and Merrylees (2009) NHS HEE Toolkit (Longstaff 2012)

useful benchmark against which to evaluate learning on international placements. The KSF focuses on six dimensions:

1. Communication
2. Personal and people development

3. Health, safety and security[3]
4. Service Improvement
5. Quality
6. Equality and Diversity

The following sections present the survey and interview findings under the headings outlined in Fig. 3.1.

## KNOWLEDGE AND SKILLS

Perhaps the most obvious and tangible perceived benefit associated with international placements concerns the acquisition of new knowledge and skills. Indeed, for many, this may be the 'make-or-break' component under-lining any justification for embedding such placements within higher educa-tion curricula (and committing resource to them). Drawing on the distinction between explicit and tacit skills (above) we have distinguished two components to this. Firstly, we discuss the acquisition of new knowl-edge. This includes both clinical and technical skills directly linked to the students' curricula and future profession and more foundational areas of knowledge about contexts, systems and resource management. We then move on to discuss the more operational dimension facilitating translation of knowledge into useable skills.

## SYSTEMS THINKING

One of the areas students commonly referred to in terms of new knowledge could be loosely described as systems thinking. Students working in a narrow pocket of a large complex organisation (such as the NHS) often find it difficult to step back and consider the system as a whole. Spending time in a low resource setting where systems are malfunctioning is so very tangible that it forces students to engage in systems thinking as a component of problem–solving (see below). And, in the process of this, and from their position outside of the NHS they are then able to reflect on the NHS *as a system*.

Knowledge of how other health systems operate (Murdoch-Eaton and Green 2011) and experiencing different clinical environments (Dowell

---

[3] This is the only area that does not map directly onto identified learning out-comes. However, this forms a key focus of placement organisation in the EEPs.

and Merrylees 2009) are often cited amongst the motivations for students to undertake elective placements and also as potential outcomes of them. Of the EEP students surveyed, 57% believed their placement had a very strong impact and 29% believed that their placement had strong impact on their learning regarding systems thinking. Some students felt that the insight gained through being placed in an unfamiliar context was illuminating in terms of facilitating their understanding of healthcare systems and different ways of working to those in the UK:

> It gave me a really good insight into health care systems abroad and different ways you know, the different methods that they use to do things. I thought it was really interesting to see how health care's developed . . . and sort of the managerial aspects of the hospital 'cos it was run very differently to the way we run a hospital, so that was very interesting. (Nurse, India)

This student's experience while on placement also influenced her thinking about the status of the nursing profession in different cultural and clinical contexts. Through reflective questioning of the challenges and assumptions of practices she identified the seemingly paradoxical relationship between gender, nursing and status, where nurses in India were very highly trained and respected, yet were not able to utilise their clinical skills in practice:

> I think nursing is viewed very differently over there to what it is here, and so I think they've got a lot of advancements to make in terms of autonomy and decision making. They [nurses] don't get the credit they deserve, self-esteem is very low. But that's very much a gender thing and a hierarchy sort of issue. Nursing is very low down, they have a lot more clinical skills than we are taught but they are not even allowed to dress wounds. (Nurse, India)

Other students commented on the way systems and practices operated in their placement organisation comparing this with the UK. Some went beyond simple learning to demonstrate 'epistemic humility' (Hanson et al. 2013), noting how the availability of resources and organisational hierarchies significantly influenced practice:

> We didn't want to be too intrusive, and tell them that that this is how they should do things because a lot of the ways that we would have done things used resources they didn't have. It is quite difficult having to take a step back and having a lot of listening and watching and not stepping in. It was quite a hierarchical system there. (Prosthetics & Orthotics, Uganda)

Some students were able to reflect and apply the learning gained while on placement to a deeper understanding of nursing practice in the UK, and were able to make improvements to their own ways of working on return. This highlights how reflective observation gained within one context can allow learning from concrete experiences to be applied to another:

> I think about it all the time when I'm on placements [in the UK]. It's just so different; we're all patient centred, patient focused, whereas over there it's more like task focused, like get the job done. And I mean, don't get me wrong, I think a lot of nurses over here can get like that too, when your workload is so big you can be like: 'Oh, you know we need to get this done, this done and this done' and when you're busy you know it can be like that, but I think that's what it's taught me as well, try to take your time with your patient and just explain what you're doing and, you know just have a chat and things like that. (Nurse, India)

For some students, being in a different context and experiencing different ways of working and learning from healthcare professionals facilitated a more questioning mind-set on return:

> I think we learnt more from them, definitely the really good nurses and doctors, more from them than they have learnt from us. They were showing us things, the procedures and such. There's not really much over there that we see over here, it's completely different . . . I think it is really useful to see that 'cos it makes you come back and question why you do things in a certain way. (Nurse, Uganda)

It is clear from the evaluation that simply being outside of the system you are accustomed to and have been weaned in generates a capacity for systems thinking both in the host setting but also in relation to the UK NHS. And this form of learning applied to some degree in both hands-on (EEP) and observational-only (India) placements. One component of this system concerns management of scarce resources.

## RESOURCE AWARENESS

Awareness of resource use and resourcing of healthcare is an important learning outcome of international placements (Brookfield 1995; Elit et al. 2011; Murdoch-Eaton and Green 2011). From the post-placement survey, 74% and 14% respectively believed their placement had a very strong or strong impact on their resource awareness. Many students expressed shock and surprise at the lack of resources in the host countries:

> I'm going from having all of your staff, equipment, tools and everything and going a month without it and then going back to it – it is a real shock. (Mental Health nurse, Uganda)

> We've got the resources whereas they don't. Sometimes they just wouldn't have the medication in stock and that's just the way it is. If it wasn't in stock and the family couldn't afford certain medications, they'd just go without it, so that was quite tough. (Nurse, Uganda)

Some students were able to make direct links between the lack of resources in their placement setting to (global) structural inequality, and how this constrains the agency of healthcare workers:

> The main challenge I saw in every clinic, workshop and teaching syllabus is the lack of resources. I know this is due to the lack of money available to the hospital and very little can be done to change this in the present economic state. (Prosthetics/Orthotics, Uganda)

Through concrete experience of the constraints in Uganda, students identified the challenges faced by healthcare workers and demonstrated an awareness of how these impacted upon practice. This was particularly marked in disciplines like prosthetics which rely quite heavily on materials:

> I have been able to experience first-hand the numerous challenges encountered in a low-resource healthcare setting. It is clear that the greatest issue here is access to materials and machinery. (Prosthetics & Orthotics, Uganda)

In the following case, a nursing student describes the lack of consumables and equipment that are essential to the effective performance of even the most basic nursing in Uganda:

> One of my biggest challenges was the lack of resources that they had. This included equipment, gloves, medication and fluids. The lack of resources was not really overcome as we just had to work with what we had. I was fortunate that I had brought my own stethoscope and sphygmomanometer from home so I took that with me during my placement. (Nurse, Uganda)

Although, as in the case described above, the lack of resources made it hard to perform even the most basic of tasks, others indicated that being in a low resource setting made them very conscious of how wasteful practices in the UK often were, and through this concrete experience, tacit knowledge and subsequent reflection, they changed their way of thinking about practice in the UK. This level of resource awareness also developed on observational placements in India but without the intensity of personal frustration:

> They don't have the advanced equipment we have...they need the same equipment like we do. Because, at the end of the day they are patients as well. They are people so it's quite sad that we have all this technology. We probably waste so much. And they don't waste anything; they use everything they have. If we used less we could send it over there or to Africa. Or, to other countries where they need them. (Nurse, India)

These comments are interesting as they highlight the risk that students may generalise their experiences to caricature wider Indian or Ugandan health systems as facing severe resource and technology constraints when of course both countries have private sector hospitals with state of the art technology. This underlines the importance of reflective practice and having experienced mentors in country and on their return to the UK to frame and challenge the students' immediate experiences and systems thinking. Also, perhaps to encourage students to consider the practical impacts of donations. Nevertheless, in the context of NHS financial crisis, their experiences foster an acute awareness of waste:

> I look at practice in a different way. I'm very conscious of the waste we produce now and the sort of the practice that we have. We're a bit nonchalant about things so I think it's been really good in that respect because you're very mindful of what you're using and whether you definitely need that or not. (Nurse, India)

Another student echoes this sentiment:

> I learnt that people in the NHS take things for granted. I learnt that even though they had limited resources they made the most of what they had and in the NHS they waste so much. (Nurse, India)

## CLINICAL AND TECHNICAL SKILLS

Clinical knowledge and skills have been identified as key learning attributes during electives (Dowell and Merrylees 2009). Practically all of the students felt that they had acquired clinical and practice-based knowledge, or technical skills (Williams 2006; Williams and Balatz 2008). Of the EEP students surveyed; 28%, 26% and 32% respectively thought their placements had a very strong, strong or moderate impact on their skills and competence. In many cases they spoke of having access to more specialist skills in their field or at the margins of their field that they have difficulty accessing during placements in the UK.

As we explained in Chapter 1, the India placements were organised via HEE on an observation-only basis whereas students in Uganda had the opportunity to practice, under supervision. The learning outcomes (in terms of clinical skills) are quite different. Students undertaking hands-on clinical placements reported intense and accelerated learning (Norton and Marks-Moran 2014; Stephens 2015). The following example is typical:

> It was an experience and a half, I loved it. We did so much. I did more in those four weeks than I did in my whole first year and learned more in those four weeks than my first year. (Nurse, Uganda)

In the next case the occupational therapy student was able to gain key paediatric experience during her Ugandan placement:

> It was good to get some paediatric experience, that was amazing because I don't think I would be able to get that experience [in the UK] because when you go to do something like that they want previous experience so that broke a bit of a barrier. (Occupational Therapist, Uganda)

Respondents used the concepts of 'exposures' or 'spoking-out' to identify unique learning encounters that they would not have had the opportunity to experience in the UK. Adult nursing students had the opportunity to work with babies or gain exposure to maternity cases, for example, which they had not had access to at home:

> I've never really done [observations] on babies so being able to monitor them and see how they care for them. (Nurse, Uganda)

> I gained some clinical skills even doing clinical observations. Also the maternity side of things, I would never have otherwise known. (Nurse, Uganda)

> I had lots of personal achievements. I assisted in the delivery of twins and 3 little girls. I took part in cervical screening which was an amazing experience and I was part of the hand hygiene training at Bukuuku health centre. (Nurse, Uganda)

Our ethnographic experience of working alongside students on placement, backed up by their interviews, suggests that placements in the UK are often quite narrowly defined in line with the specialisms they are working towards and students have limited opportunity to see beyond these and experience work at the interface of professional boundaries. This does not imply that the skills they gain are irrelevant. In some cases, students explained how the experience had influenced their future career ambitions perhaps involving a shift in emphasis. In other examples students referred to the value of this more holistic learning when they came to have placements in accident and emergency contexts (for example). In such environments, an adult nurse may well be faced with a pregnant mother or a child. Paramedic students who also spent time in health centres dealing primarily with maternity cases and children spoke of the value of this more multi-disciplinary learning to their future roles and the confidence it had given them to manage such cases. The broader exposure to cases that a student may not have immediate access to in the UK was also mentioned by mental-health nurses in Uganda who worked both at the very hard end of institutionalised and highly medicated patients and in community out-reach work:

> In terms of mental health specifically, I've learned more about variation in diagnosis and how it can manifest and present differently. My placements so far [in the UK] had been quite stable and I just had to discharge patients, but there I could see crisis situations, which was quite an eye-opener. Eventually I will have to assess people in these conditions so it's given me knowledge of that. (Paramedic, Uganda)

In addition to this 'spoking out' most students in the Uganda placements referred to the level of access they had to more complex and emergency cases in their area of specialism. This was often related in their interviews to the issue of responsibility and confidence as the knowledge they had learnt from lectures and textbooks could now be applied in practice:

> It has been invaluable to gain such varied clinical exposure and to have been given a level of access and responsibility that is beyond anything we have experienced in the UK... The hands-on exposure has allowed us to build upon our practical skills through assessing and providing patients with relevant treatments. (Prosthetics & Orthotics, Uganda)

The same comments would doubtless be found amongst students who had taken part in traditional unsupervised electives and we are acutely aware of the line here between giving students access to cases that whilst presenting unique learning opportunities could challenge their competency. It is important to emphasise that all of the students in Uganda were supervised by both Ugandan and UK professionals and were not operating on their own.

Students were able to reflect on this new learning both in terms of clinical skills but also critical thinking. In the following case a prosthetics student suggests that this has contributed to her development as a rounded professional:

> This placement was a great opportunity for me to develop my knowledge and develop skills required to become a more rounded and efficient healthcare practitioner. The clinical exposure allowed here in Uganda was almost incomparable to those received in the course so far in the UK. Being in a developing country also increases the amount of critical thinking required to fulfil a job role of an orthotist or prosthetist... Going during this aspect of our studies has been extremely beneficial in terms of clinical exposure and I have learnt a tremendous amount of information, skills etc. (Prosthetics & Orthotics, Uganda)

In the final example in this section the nursing student reflects on the value of her learning to her wider professional role. However, she also makes an important point; that the placement enhanced some skills but did not cover all aspects of her 'skills book':

> On reflection it has made me a better nurse not because I've seen any wild animal attacks or rare diseases. I didn't work on all of the skills from my skills book but I did work on getting the basics of care right. I realised how important it is to monitor the small changes in patients and how crucial documentation is to understand how the patient is progressing. (Nurse, Uganda)

In this case, she emphasises the back-to-basics quality of her learning rather than the exotic learning she may have anticipated. Certainly, it is these skills that she will now be utilising in her placements in the UK. Her point about not working on all the skills is important however. It is much more difficult in a low resource setting to ensure a comprehensive skills enhancement in line with any UK curriculum and this has implications in terms of skills mapping and potential augmentation on return. This would certainly be the case if the skills map included working with specific forms of equipment, for example. A number of students explained how the clinical exposure helped develop their self-awareness and shape or confirmed their future career aspirations:

> I've learnt more in that month in Uganda than the four months on my placement in the UK. I want to work in adult mental health. (Social Work, Uganda)

> It has definitely been beneficial to my course and to what I want to do in future ... It has made me put a specific thing in a bigger picture. We have to look at those things in our course but we've never had to deal with it practically, until we went out there. (Business studies, Uganda)

In our sister book on the learning of professional Volunteers, we noted the contribution that placements made to confidence in using existing skills (Ackers et al. 2017). Most of the students on the EEP placements spoke of their new-found confidence in their clinical skills. The idea of 'deliberative practice' is associated with a particular theory of learning that emphasises the value of repeated engagement with a particular skill or skill set (Ericsson et al. 1993). In our work on the gains associated with professional voluntarism, we noted the gains that NHS professionals experienced through repeated exercise of pre-existing skills (Ackers et al. 2017). This dimension of learning was also in evidence amongst the students on clinical placements in Uganda.

> I feel a bit more confident if something happened to be able to actually resuscitate a baby. (Nurse, Uganda)

> It's given me an awful lot of confidence. I thought I was quite confident any way but it enhanced my confidence to step forward in the skills I use in the UK. (Nurse, Uganda)

In the final case the nursing student explains how this had an immediate impact on her professional practice in the UK:

> Confidence was the most important thing. I went back to accident and emergency and I was just so much more confident; when emergencies came in I didn't lose my cool, I had a lot more calm after being there because we dealt with lots of emergencies. I wasn't as panicky because I had been in that situation before. (Nurse, Uganda)

## PERSONAL VALUES AND THE PATIENT INTERFACE

We noted above the focus on equality and diversity in the NHS Knowledge and Skills framework and the emphasis of personal values and value systems in the literature on international placements (Brookfield 1995; Elit et al. 2011). For convenience, the following section distinguishes learning directly related to personal values from that concerning wider social values although of course the two are intrinsically related.

The Francis Report (2013) emphasised the importance of care and compassion at all levels of the NHS workforce. This stimulated a drive toward a 'value-based' strategy (Waugh et al. 2014) which has placed the '6 Cs'; Care, Compassion, Competence, Communication, Courage and Commitment (NHS 2016) at the heart of the skills enhancement agenda. In addition to the more explicit clinical skills identified above respondents identified a wide range of less tangible skills and knowledge acquired on placements. These included both personal and professional development and again, embodied tacit rather than explicit (or technical) knowledge (Williams 2006).

Through concrete experience augmented through reflection and self-evaluation, students identified care and compassion as important components of their clinical practice. 57% and 32% respectively stated that their placement had a very strong or strong impact on their perception of compassion and the importance of empathy. The following comment is typical:

> In terms of nursing, it just highlighted to me how important it is to have that relationship with your patient and to just to be reassuring and things like that because there is nothing worse than when you feel like no one really cares about you, when you're ill. (Nurse, India)

For some students on observational placements in India, this profound experience coupled with their inability to intervene and assist if a patient was in pain caused some anxiety:

> You're not used to seeing patients that are like severely in pain, severely distressed and that in itself is just really hard to deal with and you don't, you're never prepared for that because that's just not something that you would see here. And obviously as a nurse you want to look after people and you want to do your best to care for people and make them more comfortable and settled and you feel like you can't do that for them, and you're like, what am I here for? What's the point, what am I doing? You're just making a dent in it you know, you're not making a difference. (Nurse, India)

As we have explained (in Chapter 1) the India placements were not a part of the Ethical Education Placements Model and our experience of them as observation-only placements has lead us to question their impact on student learning and, perhaps more significantly, their compliance with ethical principles. Having said that, students on clinical placements will also experience a sense of disempowerment at the lack of resources and human resource context and the impact this has on their ability to demonstrate care and compassion:

> Throughout my three years [at university] everything that they've taught us is all about the patient, caring for the patient and having empathy and sympathy and you know looking after their needs ... once you're out there you just see people dying of reasons that you could literally treat them with no problem over here. (Nurse, Uganda)

> It touched me a bit because there was a lot of preventable death over there, people just died but if they were over here probably wouldn't have died ... you feel a bit helpless. (Nurse, Uganda)

Many students found being in a different setting challenging and some felt that systems themselves thwarted practice and their ability to provide appropriate levels of care. It is quite different to witness an absolute lack of resources as opposed to an apparent systems failure resulting in inefficient use or abuse of resources. In the following case the nursing student interpreted the situation as a lack of care on the part of Ugandan health workers:

In some situations it just seemed as if people didn't really care. If someone was in a lot of pain and they were asking for pain medications, they were like: 'No, the [medicines] round isn't until this evening they'll be fine', you know not really caring that much and obviously nursing is a caring profession. (Nurse, Uganda)

For others, experiencing different systems challenged their own world view. Being aware of the conditions and constraints host systems operated in allowed them to place their worldview in context, and realise that practice is framed by context;

There were only two doctors working different shifts, so I think a lot can't be helped. They try to do the best they can but it could easily be much better, there's no dignity or respect. (Nurse, Uganda)

In other cases, students experienced situations that, in themselves, did not reflect resource shortages in any simple sense. In the following case in India, a midwifery student observed a lack of attention to privacy or consent:

Women had no privacy, even in the antenatal there was more than one woman per room and there was no curtain or anything and it was hard to sleep . . . and also the fact that they didn't have to consent to anything, the doctors just did it, although they may have consented but we didn't know, it could have been the language or culture, but it's just second nature to do that here. They also took the baby away straight away, just to make sure it was ok, but it was in a different room. So they didn't get much chance to bond, the baby was just left crying. (Midwife, India)

The historical legacy and enduring effects of structural inequality between high and low resource settings and the differences in positionalities of students from high-income countries[4] and populations in low-income countries means that there can be assumptions of superiority (Elit et al. 2011). Additionally, 'benevolent imperialism' (Huish 2012) and hubris[5]

---

[4] It is important to point out that many of the students on placement were themselves from diverse backgrounds including students of African or Asian descent.

[5] Defined as dangerous overconfidence.

(Hanson et al. 2011) can characterise the perceptions and interactions of students:

> The main problem really is their culture and their beliefs ... I'd say it makes you appreciate people's dignity much more, because over there they don't do that over there, there's no dignity or respect. It makes you more aware of different cultures. (Nurse, Uganda)

Once they had time to reflect on their experiences, some students recalibrated their initial perceptions of staff in host organisations and were able to place their actions in context:

> It's mad because I remember thinking 'Oh my god the way they are doing that is so bad; that is terrible' but actually it's not. Now I've come home and thought about it, that's just how they cope, that's how they deal with such low resources and you know those people are still being treated as best as they can be. It's not bad, it's just they are doing what they can with what they've got. But for us, at first it's shocking. (Nurse, India)

Some students referred to what they perceived as a lack of motivation of healthcare workers in their placement setting.[6] Again, this was something that had been raised with them prior to undertaking placements in Uganda and most were able to place the behaviour of individuals within a particular structural context, recognising that people's apparent motivation would be shaped by extrinsic factors and the way that systems operate:

> Motivation wise that's a big issue of course in Uganda, we went to lectures about motivation and absenteeism. That's part of it I'm sure – other reasons as well – but lower motivation because obviously people would be thinking I'm doing the work of more than two or three people and they are not here. Obviously it affects the motivation, they could be overworked which results in them not going to work and it could snowball out of control. (Nurse, Uganda)

---

[6] Health-worker motivation has formed the basis of much of our project work in Uganda. Students attended a workshop on this in June 2016 involving local health workers and senior managers. The impact of motivation on health-worker behaviour is discussed in Ackers and Ackers-Johnson (2016).

These examples emphasise the continuing impact of placements and the important learning that happens post return as students reflect upon and make sense of their experience. Harnessing this and facilitating discussion within peer groups optimises the learning of the individuals concerned and enables it to spread to others. It also provides the opportunity to challenge and reduce the risks that students will draw general and perhaps essentialised conclusions from their immersions. Many of the students felt that their experiences abroad made them aware and appreciative of their privilege in the UK, in terms of available resources and the treatment that patients were able to receive:

> There's a lot of people suffering in the hospital which is quite difficult because there weren't many beds, it made you appreciate what we have here. (Prosthetics & Orthotics, Uganda)

Unsurprisingly, the experience of observing or working in a low resource setting encouraged all students to reflect on the role that the UK's National Health Service plays in providing access to health care on a universal basis irrespective of a patient's ability to pay:

> It confirmed how privileged our life is and how precious the NHS is. It was heart-breaking to see a young mum of 20 die for the lack of an antibiotic given on time. (Nurse, Uganda)

This regard for the NHS extends to an awareness of the expertise and commitment of NHS staff – whose cadres they are soon to join – giving them confidence in their own career decision making:

> I've got a new-found appreciation for our nurses and the hard work they put in and the level of care that we provide. Everyone slags off the NHS...you have no idea how lucky you are to have been born in this country, receive the level of healthcare that we receive. Halfway across the world it is a very very different story, and they're so grateful for the care they receive. They don't complain in comparison to [the UK] where like everybody loves to moan. (Prosthetics & Orthotics, Uganda)

The example cited above exemplifies one of the outcomes of placements that we also discussed in our evaluation of professional voluntarism (Ackers and Ackers-Johnson 2016); namely reflection on the attitudes of

NHS users. The effect that placements in low resource settings have on reinforcing a commitment to care and compassion goes hand-in-hand with a reflection on the lack of appreciation of many patients in the UK and the demands they place on hard-pressed staff:

> It was a massive culture shock going to India, but an even bigger one coming home. I remember being on the ward and a patient was shouting at a nurse because she had given him the wrong meal and he was saying how crap the NHS was, telly wasn't working so he was discharging himself etc. And I just remember thinking, you should be thankful, you've got a bed, clean bedding, I didn't say anything but I thought it. (Nurse, India)

It is important that opportunities are given within the curriculum for students returning from placements to make sense of these sometimes conflicting feelings to understand what care and compassion means in different settings and how to handle such patients. In this way, through reflective questioning of both the challenges and assumptions of practices, students demonstrated an increased understanding of different value systems (Brookfield 1995; Elit et al. 2011; Murdoch-Eaton and Green 2011).

The sense of frustration or helplessness that students experience can extend to trauma particularly when students witness deaths. All of the child nurses working on the neonatal units in Fort Portal experienced neonatal deaths and other students experienced maternal deaths. Students were also upset by the very different approaches to death in Uganda. It is important that all parties involved in educational placements in low resource settings are prepared for the level of trauma involved and find ways of managing expectations and experiences of this from induction processes through placement supervision and during their return to study. Perhaps the most important component of this is the provision of supervision by UK professional volunteers on the ground who are able to mentor and support the students. Whilst exposure to death and to cultural differences in the treatment of dead patients can be highly traumatic, this is also an important source of learning for students that they are often insulated from in the UK. It is all too easy, faced with the immediate exposure to death, to judge patients and health workers and find them lacking in care and compassion:

> It was horrible. There was a dead baby on the floor one day. But it was kind of good that we were exposed because that can never happen here . . . there is no compassion over there; that was one of the hardest things coz when one

of the babies died, and the doctors saw them dead, there was no grief, no compassion, no emotion, it was just really cold. So it was a learning part for me that I will never do it like that. (Nurse, Uganda)

This case takes us interesting another area of critical learning for students; typically referred to as 'cultural competence'.

## CULTURAL COMPETENCE

The introduction to this book referred to the impact of globalisation on UK universities. The forces of globalisation and internationalisation have and continue to have a massive impact on the National Health Service both as an employer and service provider. Perhaps the most immediate example of this concerns global labour markets in terms of both exporting UK professions and importing their foreign peers. Staff shortages have been commonplace within the UK National Health Service since its creation and it has responded to these through international recruitment.[7] The NHS has a code of practice on international recruitment from low resource settings which aims to reduce the damaging effects of 'brain drain':

> Any international recruitment of healthcare professionals should not prejudice the healthcare systems of developing countries. Healthcare professionals should not be actively recruited from developing countries, unless there is a Government-to-Government agreement to support recruitment activities.[8]

In practice this code seems to have done little to prevent the leakage of large volumes of health workers from low resource settings into the NHS. Whilst these trends are common throughout the world, the UK is one of the biggest importers of foreign health workers. A report by the Organisation for Economic Co-operation and Development (OECD 2015) has shown that 35% of NHS doctors were born abroad, putting Britain ahead of every

---

[7] There is not scope in this book to comment on the wider ethical dynamics of these processes but for discussion.

[8] http://www.nhsemployers.org/your-workforce/recruit/employer-led-recruitment/international-recruitment/uk-code-of-practice-for-international-recruitment

other country in the European Union except Luxembourg. The same report highlighted a sharp increase in the number of foreign born nurses working in the UK NHS, rising from 15.2% in 2001/2002 to 21.7% in 2011/2012. It explains how, within this same decade, 40% of the overall growth in the number of doctors and 65% of the growth in the number nurses can be attributed to the arrival of foreign workers. Many of these foreign workers come from low- and middle-income countries; for example in England as at 30 September 2015, there were 18,096 NHS Hospital and Community Health Services staff from India, 479 from Uganda, 4,142 from Zimbabwe, 5,124 from Nigeria and 13,533 from the Philippines amongst many other countries (NHS Digital 2016)

Not only has the composition of the NHS undergone a transformation but wider society has become far more diverse and multicultural than ever before. OECD figures from 2013 estimated that 12.3% of the UK population were 'foreign born', equating to over 7.8 million people. The differing demographic, socioeconomic and cultural backgrounds lead to differing health needs which must be catered for by the National Health Service. In order for this to happen, staff require additional skill, competency and experience to deal with the less familiar and potentially more complex patient cases. Macfarlane and Dorkenoo (2015) examine the example of female genital mutilation (FGM), estimating that the number of women aged 15–49 with FGM born in countries in which FGM is practised but living in England and Wales had increased from an estimated 66,000 in 2001 to 103,000 in 2011. They attribute this increase largely to immigration to the UK from African nations where FGM is commonplace such as Somalia, Egypt, Guinea and Djibouti. The rise in cases of FGM has prompted widespread health policy review and staff guidelines and training recommendations (Topping 2015). Other similar cases can be found in terms of the prevalence of infectious diseases, such as HIV and Tuberculosis, for which rates are higher for non-UK-born people. In terms of mental health, Raphaely and O'Moore (2010) concluded that higher rates of depression and anxiety exist among refugees and asylum seekers than the national population or other categories of migrants.

These trends highlight a large and expanding international workforce and a complex, diversifying range of patients within the UK National Health Service. In many ways, professionals from all over the world are working alongside UK health staff to treat patients from all over the world. This leads to greater demands in areas such as workforce integration, cultural awareness and sensitivity, competency and human resource management. It also requires staff to have additional skills in the areas of communication and teaching to allow for effective cooperation and the exchange of knowledge, skills and capabilities in the workplace. This is the context within which the development of ethical educational placements is taking place.

In the introduction we questioned whether it is possible for students to unproblematically become 'culturally aware' or develop 'cultural competence' through merely participating in international placements. Practically all of the students mentioned culture, usually in relation to difference, in terms of different systems, ways of working and values. Our survey suggested that 78% and 18% of students respectively believed their placement had a very strong or strong impact on their cultural awareness.

Returning to the discussion above about death, some students were able to reflect on their experiences from the perspective of cultural differences rather than concluding simplistically that Ugandans lacked compassion. In the following case, the nursing student recognised the complex relationships between human emotions and outward displays of grief:

> The women, when they are having babies and in pain, they just get on with it. There was one woman who was basically just smiling at me the whole way through her labour, she looked so beautiful as well and I just thought oh my god! But then there was one baby who was going to die and when the mum was told she didn't show a massive amount of emotion. I don't know if it's because that's so common to them it was just quite strange to see. (Nurse, Uganda)

Another nursing student describes witnessing the death of a baby in Uganda:

> One of the challenges I faced was the lack of emotion people show when they have a baby or if somebody passes away. I found this very challenging especially when somebody passed away. I could not understand how they did not cry. I overcame this by learning that it is part of their culture not to show any emotion and they often do that in private. (Nurse, Uganda)

Some students were positive about the differences they witnessed, demonstrating epistemic humility through highlighting aspects which they felt were lacking in the UK. By way of example, many recognised the role played by the extended family and the wider community in supporting patients. This was evident across a number of disciplines and in both the observation-only (India) and hands-on (Uganda) placements. In the first case reported here the paramedic student spoke of the importance of family to patients in Uganda:

> I was able to witness how much family assistance with care is relied on, and the generosity of members of the public towards those without families to help their recovery. (Paramedic, Uganda)

Similar comments were made by a midwifery student involved in the India placement who mentioned the support provided by family members reflecting on how this would be handled in the UK:

> In India they have the whole family sleeping in the corridor waiting for them. In our hospital we don't even let them wait in the waiting room when their daughter's in labour, they have to do down stairs to Costa ... So the difference is just mad, and like for that woman it could be completely reassuring having mum and dad there. (Midwife, India)

The student in this case is clearly considering some of the potential benefits of having family in the delivery room. She does not reflect at this point on some of the potential risks associated with this in terms of infection prevention or the privacy of other patients; these are issues that could form the basis of interesting discussion about care in context and the boundaries of individual freedom on return to the UK. Others highlighted how family members were kept informed about patients which enabled them to play a meaningful role in supporting their care once discharged from hospital. One of the mental-health students placed in Uganda explains how the family are more engaged in the care of their family members:

> I think there was a lot more family involvement in Uganda like in the mental health unit than in the UK [where] you tend to treat the person. In Uganda they connect with the family member to look after them so you got the chance to explain to the family member what condition it is and how it impacts them so that they understand better so I think some of the families in Uganda understood the conditions better than sometimes here because

they never really get that information from a healthcare professional, so that was good. (Nurse, Uganda)

Social work students on community placements in Uganda were also very positive about the role of the wider community in supporting vulnerable members and reflected on how this approach could be beneficial to the UK:

> I did learn a lot, the community projects that are there are something that I haven't seen as much of in the UK, there seems to be a lot more community enterprise there. (Social Worker, Uganda)

The social work student in the next case talks about the 'Goats for Life' project aimed at developing social enterprise to enable families to pull themselves out of poverty. While the project itself is unlikely to take roots in the UK context, his reference to the growth of individualism in the UK is immediately relevant to his future role as a social worker:

> One of the projects was the Goats for Life project... So we went to the market and bought 4 or 5 goats and delivered them out to the community. Seeing the wider family network and how that goat can bring them all together was good, because everyone came round and everyone was involved, which was lovely to see. You knew that there was a bond there, and with the child there that had no parents. People would help the child get to school and things and people helped the grandmother out, and I think that's important skills to learn. Right now [in the UK] things are stuck behind doors, and we don't know problems with our own neighbours, and I think it's really important for social workers to learn that community can exist, even if that's in Africa. Were taught not to see it, and that individuality is the trump card, but it is good to see a different way, and see how it can be good to work together. This is a community coming together to help. (Social Worker, Uganda)

In the final case another social work student describes the emphasis on community in Uganda as 'progressive':

> I consider the community social work method which I have experienced in Uganda as very progressive, effective and efficient. (Social Worker, Uganda)

It may come as a shock to many to see social work in Uganda described in such positive terms. One of the social science students similarly described a local midwifery-lead health centre as fitting perfectly with her own personal commitment to natural child birth and rejection of the medicalisation of maternity services in the UK (as she saw it). It would be useful to work through these perceptions with students on return to understand what lies behind them, not as a criticism of Ugandan systems but rather to develop a deeper critique. Community social work, 'natural' childbirth and the involvement of families in mental health may be necessary responses to fundamental gaps in systems; the lack of public services as much as attention to cultural differences. Nevertheless, these observations provide the basis for critical reflection and learning.

Although we question whether just being in a different context builds culturally competence, for some students, having the experience of being in a different setting gave them knowledge of a different country, culture and environment and engender confidence about difference. In the following example a mental-health student suggests that the immersive nature of her experience in Uganda will support her future practice in what is a very multi-cultural environment:

> I felt I came back and got more understanding of the different cultures because Liverpool's really diverse; you get a lot of different patients from all around the world and I feel like I can sympathise with them a lot more and understand them a bit more. (Nurse, Uganda)

It is interesting to reflect on this case as the student is deeply embedded in a very diverse home environment; far more diverse in fact that the one she experienced in Uganda. We would argue that it is as much the students' experiences of being an outsider in Uganda or India that hones this experience as it is the exposure to cultural difference per se. The effect of the placements on students' awareness of culture was evident both in the Indian and Ugandan contexts. Echoing previous discussion about the role of family in health care the following student reflects on her placement in India:

> It's made me a better nurse because the UK is becoming more multi-cultural so I have to – not that it's a bad thing – I have to face different cultures and to be able to experience their culture and what they normally do. The patients' family come in to wash them, to feed them [in India] whereas here the healthcare systems do that, the nurses do that care. So if they felt

more comfortable with the family, if it was appropriate, we would encourage the family to come in to offer that care. That's what I would like to do if I was running a ward. (Nurse, India)

Clearly there are many reasons why this approach is both necessary in India and Uganda as these roles are not considered a part of normal health worker roles and would present real challenges to the NHS, in terms of privacy and infection prevention control. Once again experiences such as these and the critical thinking they provoke provide fertile ground for discussion with peers on return rather than immediately transportable policy options.

In the spirit of epistemic humility, having particular concrete experiences and being able to reflect on them and conceptually abstract such experiences, gave some students the opportunity to reconsider how they would practice in the future, in terms of how they would relate to both colleagues and patients:

I wasn't too aware of understanding people and the differences they have due to culture and religions and. I think just having a bit more knowledge . . . if I was to obviously care for a patient who was of a different religion or culture I think I would probably take the time to go away and actually learn a bit more about it and to be able to understand them a little bit better like in that sense. (Nurse, Uganda)

The midwifery student in the following case reflects on her experience of observing mothers in India and explains how this has enabled her to understand Indian women's attitudes towards breast feeding in the UK:

We learnt a lot of cultural stuff. Now I can understand why Indian women sometimes act the way they do here. They're not rude, that's just how they are and their culture and they're not used to us being friendly. I've come across a few Indian patients here and I've just accepted this is what they want rather than saying that's just how we do it here. They tend to bottle feed the first 3 days, just because of their culture. Before I would tell them not to – now I just accept that's how they are. (Midwife, India)

Once again this raises points for discussion with her tutors and peer group; it may be that from a professional perspective simply accepting bottle feeding is deemed inappropriate or out of line with public health protocols in the UK. Witnessing cultural difference does not necessarily mean accepting all forms of behaviour but it does help to understand what lies behind that behaviour. The following example represents similar points for discussion:

> To put it into context, I was working on a ward (back home in the UK) and there was an Indian lady having surgery and there was a lot of her family around her bed, like a lot, which you see in India because that's their culture. But I remember a few of the care staff where like 'oh no we can't have that many relatives, oh my god no they've got to go' and it was only because I had been to India and I knew that that's what happens there and that's their culture and it sounds bad but I said to my colleagues it will make it easier for you because they want to look after their relative whilst they are a patient so let them and you just be in the background if they need anything. (Nurse, India)

The nursing student in the next case talks about how the awareness she has gained in India will help her relationships with Indian health workers:

> A massive thing I gained in cultural awareness, both for patients and also there are a lot of Indian nurses coming over here and now I feel I have a better relationship with them. To be honest, I used to think they were lazy, because they didn't do personal care but now I know they don't do it and sometimes you'd ask them and they would just look at you and not do it. So now, I just don't ask them now and it's not that they are doing anything wrong it's just how they are taught and it's their culture. And I know you can say they should work within the NMC [Nursing and Midwifery Council] code of conduct but India has given me that awareness of how to deal with that stuff. (Nurse, India)

The students' conclusion that it is OK for nursing students from India not to engage in personal care is quite alarming. Certainly it is essential that foreign staff in the NHS work to the same protocols as their UK peers but understanding these cultural dynamics and global differences within the mixed economy of care is critical to encouraging individual behaviour change.

Finally, a number of students emphasised how the cultural learning they had engaged in was in fact a two-way process. Examples of sharing information, knowledge exchange and developing understanding of how different contexts and systems operate appeared to be key:

> I'd say definitely like culture-wise, they gained things because they would ask all sorts of questions about what it's like, like what we think and stuff like

that, especially our buddie learnt loads about what it's like over here because she was asking us so many questions and stuff... We learnt as much as they did really, because we'd just swap the stories. (Midwife, India)

## COMMUNICATION

The enhancement of communication skills is identified in much of the existing research on learning outcomes (Jeffrey et al. 2011). In our survey, 40% and 43% of students respectively felt that their placement had a very strong or strong impact on their communication skills, stating they were better able to adapt the way they communicated to fit with different contexts and situations. In this way, professional skills development and acquisition (communication) could be understood to link to the development of other skills (managing difficult situations):

I learnt so much not only to help me within my nursing career but I learnt a lot about different cultures and developed my communication skills and my ability to cope under stressful and difficult situations. (Nurse, Uganda)

Some students reported challenges in communicating with staff and patients, but were able to improvise in the way they communicated, demonstrating flexibility and adaptability, and recognised that developing communication skills was important for future practice:

The language barrier was a massive challenge. Most of the patients I came across could not speak English and I could not speak their language. The nurses and healthcare workers also did not speak much English. This made it very difficult when communicating as I often had to use hand gestures. (Nurse, Uganda)

When talking about communication some students demonstrated humility, awareness of privilege and difference and reflected on what it is to be in the minority or perceived as 'other':

You just sort of like get annoyed with those who don't speak English, but we got culturally aware... we were the only ones speaking English, and you were just more aware of how they must feel when they are somewhere [where nobody speaks their language]. (Nurse, Uganda)

The following podiatry student talks about her skills in non-verbal communication in Uganda:

> Obviously not everyone over there speaks English but you can still kind of communicate, with expressions in the way you behave. Sometimes you didn't know what they were saying but you could still get an idea of what they were saying by their body language and expression. (Podiatrist, Uganda)

Even where staff were speaking English the following nursing students showed an awareness of how miscommunication can arise:

> I haven't worked with any African patients since being in Uganda but I think I probably have more of an understanding of accepting, if you ask them to do something or you know the way they reply, I think I've had more patience and I know why they're saying what they are, and just try and approach the situation a bit differently but not be upset or angry at the fact they've turned around and said something completely out of order. (Nurse, Uganda)

In the following case the student nurse learns how to interpret a use of English in Uganda that she is unaccustomed to and accept this as a facet of cultural differences; her own language suggests that she continues to view this as 'wrong':

> At first you get on with it, like trying cursing under your breath but then you think well sometimes it's different cultures and the way they deal with things...sometimes people don't necessarily mean to be rude or awful, it's just how they've spoken most of their life or how they speak to people, and nobody's ever really turned around and said: you shouldn't say that to people. (Nurse, Uganda)

Other students recognised the need to modify and adapt the way they communicated to better relate to Ugandan patients. This is of particular importance in the field of mental health:

> I think it's really good...the cultural aspect of it, the communication. We used too much clinical language with the patient so they taught us how to speak to people. It was good like that. (Nurse, India)

The development of communication skills amongst students was also remarked upon by programme leads in the Universities and by Professional Volunteers:

> There was a big development of confidence, and being in a situation where people don't always speak the same language as you, or choose not to in some cases. I think it is using your communication skills in a different environment. People have mentioned things about their self-awareness of their inability to communicate . . . They learn more of the softer skills, like communication and working in a team and they learnt to assert themselves sometimes and come across in a certain way. (MMU University Programme Lead)

> They have really come together as a team and they are very good at supporting each other, and they have learnt to communicate with staff . . . it all links to the team working. (PV, Uganda)

## TEACHING AND PRESENTATION SKILLS

As we noted in Chapter 2 students undertaking placements in Uganda are given a range of potential teaching opportunities. These included contributing to teaching on the K4C sponsored degree programme in midwifery alongside our professional volunteers. They also had the opportunity to join local MMU students in social work and community development workshops and business students worked directly on joint project work as part of the hand hygiene project. This latter project involved some teaching in in local schools on basic infection prevention control. Perhaps less planned, EEP students found themselves working alongside quite large volumes of students from local colleges left to find their way without supervision in Ugandan health facilities. A number of students indicated that their placement provided them with the opportunity for personal growth and professional development, and developing teaching and presentation skills were key areas where this seemed to operate. It is apparent that such opportunities were felt to benefit future career prospects in terms of enhancing CVs, but students were also keen to make a contribution to the host setting. Some students were initially reluctant to put themselves forward, but were able to reflect on how the (concrete) experience helped their skills development. This 'learning through doing' occurred across a range of disciplines and student cohorts but was limited to those students who were involved in practice-based placements in Uganda. The respondent in the first case describes her initial reluctance to get involved in teaching:

> We didn't want to do it because we hadn't done it before and at first the students laughed at some people and it ran over quite a long time but we had chance to talk to them and have a good discussion. It also helped our presentation and teaching skills. (Social work)

In another example, paramedic students were invited to develop emergency first aid training for local ambulance drivers in Uganda who receive no training at all in this area and are not accompanied on their journeys by health professionals. In this case the students jumped at the opportunity without any reservation:

> The training we did came off well, some of the nurses came and the ambulance drivers and we were very pleased with how quickly the skills were coming on; we taught CPR and how to dress wounds and deliver babies. I think we helped a lot there because they said they do have to do a lot in the community but don't really have the training for it and I think we've been a bit of an impact there. (Paramedic, Uganda)

The prosthetic and orthotic students were given opportunities to work alongside Ugandan students in co-mentoring roles. In addition, they took part in some large group teaching:

> The opportunity arose for me to conduct an anatomy lecture discussing upper limb bony anatomy, musculature, as well as blood and nerve supply to the second year students studying orthopaedic technology. I have never had the same number of students listening to a lecture before and hence it was a great experience for me to increase confidence, reinforce my ideal subject area etc. (Prosthetics & Orthotics, Uganda)

This experience had an important confidence-building effect enabling the student to reflect positively on her own knowledge and skills base; there is nothing like teaching to make you aware of how much you know! We have already pointed to the importance of 'back-to-basics' learning in low resource settings. Students' awareness of the neglect of some of these foundational systems and skills encouraged them to engage in teaching in this area:

With a few people from my group we also did a short teaching session at Mountains of the Moon University to Nursing and Midwifery students on the importance of regular clinical observations and noticing signs of deterioration, the use of observation charts and the introduction of an Early Warning Score system. The session was quite successful and the students seemed really interested and willing to learn and change how they do things. (Nurse, Uganda)

The engagement in teaching encouraged students to see that their roles as health workers were more than simply service delivery; teaching is a core if often invisible component of everyday practice. And being aware of this supports attention to their own position as role models for other health workers:

Up until my last module at university, I never considered myself to be someone that would be seen as a teacher, yet working in Uganda made me see that as a nurse we continue to learn and teach every single day. Whether it is showing someone a small task or helping to better someone's performance of different skills. (Nurse, Uganda)

In the final case cited here a business studies student became involved in teaching large groups of students in Ugandan schools about hand hygiene:

I'll be more confidence in public speaking I won't be so shy now and I will feel more comfortable approaching complete strangers as this was challenging from the beginning but then it started to feel more normal. (Business, Uganda)

Student responses to the EEP survey were more varied regarding the impact that their placement had on their teaching and presentational skills. Fifty four percent believed their placement had a strong or very strong impact, 32% believed their placement had a moderate impact and 21% believed their placement had little or no impact. The reason for this variation is likely to be that not all students had the opportunity of engaging in university teaching or conducting presentations. The post-placement qualitative interviews however suggested students that did engage in these activities believed them to be highly beneficial to their learning.

The final section here concerns learning associated with leadership. 'Service improvement' is one of the areas identified in the NHS Knowledge and Skills framework. Service improvement is broader than leadership and may imply personal skills and values as well as influencing those of others.

## Service Improvement and Leadership Skills

As indicated above, Williams and Balatz (2008) identify management 'know-how' as a form of knowledge and management and leadership skills formed perhaps the most important element of learning amongst professional volunteers (Ackers et al. 2017). It is perhaps unsurprising that fewer students referred explicitly to management skills as something they had acquired or developed while on placement. This could reflect the early stage they were at in terms of their career, although some students were able to think ahead to how such skills could be deployed in the future. In the first example the nursing student felt empowered by her teaching role in Uganda reporting gains in confidence and communication:

> Some of the health professionals over there wanted to learn from us. A lot of it was about delegation and was teaching there, and it's quite useful coming back to the UK because it's made me a lot more confident really. Better communication, able to do management really of a ward which is what I was expecting. (Nurse, Uganda)

In the next case the nursing student suggests that the placement increased his ability to exercise autonomy:

> I think leadership and management is quite a big thing in nursing, and being able to manage myself in Uganda has helped massively. I went out there with an open mind. It's made me realise how lucky we are over here, and how well people can do with limited resources.... You are supposed to work with autonomy in nursing, and I can do that more now. (Nurse, Uganda)

Whilst relatively few students singled out management as one of the key learning outcomes, we would argue that management or leadership are composite qualities which depend heavily on other core skills embracing all of the skills discussed above. Survey responses for leadership and teamwork were very positive, with 73% of students believing their placement had a strong or very strong impact, 19% a moderate impact and 8% little impact. Responses regarding 'management skills' were weaker but still relatively positive with 59% stating a strong or very strong impact, 23% stating moderate impact and 18% stating little or no impact.

## PERSONAL GROWTH

We started this chapter with a series of quotes from students indicating the transformational quality of learning on their placements. In this final section, we return to this but in the context of what can best be described as personal growth. In many cases this was not all about new learning but about increased self-awareness and confidence at having been put to the test, immersed in an environment completely outside their previous experience and comfort zone. The EEP survey revealed that 48% of students believed their placement had a strong or very strong impact on their personal commitment and motivation, 12% stated a moderate impact and only 5% stated little or no impact. The following comment is quite typical and shows the effect of the placement in terms of what we have called 'mobility capital' increasing enthusiasm for and confidence in future mobility:

> This trip was extremely relevant to my degree. It has not only benefitted me as a mental health nurse but raised my confidence as an individual. It has inspired me to challenge myself in working outside the UK later in life. (Nurse, Uganda)

Many students spoke proactively of the impact of the placements on their future plans and were actively considering future stays in low resource settings:

> Personally, I had an absolutely brilliant time. Being a part of this Ugandan placement has only strengthened my desire to continue studies and aid research/projects that can help communities. (Prosthetics & Orthotics, Uganda)

> It is an experience that will remain with me for the rest of my life and it has confirmed my desire to go back to Africa to work in similar conditions. (Nurse, Uganda)

We referred in Chapter 1 to the fact that most if not all of the students who travelled to Uganda and India with the benefit of bursaries would not, otherwise, have had access to this kind of opportunity either for purely financial reasons or because they lacked the confidence to try to access placements. This was evident in the way many students talked about the experience of living in a foreign country with other students and away from their families for the first time:

> It's made me a different person in a sense of, because it was my first time away on my own without my family it's made me more independent, it's made me appreciate life more. (Nurse, India)

> It made you stronger as a person. It got quite emotional at times and I think being away from home as well, I've been away from home before but not for a month in a country that's completely different. Also being away from parents and family and having to make relationships with people you don't know, well you have met everyone once before but you were in that environment for 4 weeks and you kind of had to just get on. (Nurse, India)

Many students spoke of the personal journeys they had faced associated not solely with clinical exposures but with living amongst other students and outside of their comfort zones:

> It was totally different, it was like out of your comfort zone ... I was like doing things I wouldn't normally do. Like even living with a load of people that you didn't know, you've never lived with before ... I didn't think I'd cope well but I coped a lot better than I thought I would. (Nurse, Uganda)

> Well I've learned I'm even more emotional than what I think I've got, but then at the same time I'm a lot stronger than I thought I was. (Nurse, Uganda)

> My life has changed quite a lot since I've been back such as I am moving out because I feel more independent and I came back thinking maybe I should be doing more things such as going for more job opportunities and making the most of things. (Social Worker, Uganda)

> It was the worst and best thing I've ever done in my life that's all I can say. Worst in terms of it was hard, especially for me I'm just not used to that ... but the best in terms of learning about culture, health care in a different world and about myself. (Nurse, India)

> It has just made me more confident, and I now know I'd be able to go elsewhere confidently ... Definitely, it has helped with my confidence. I had an interview when I got back which I got and there were only two places so I was very pleased to get it ... I think going to Uganda made me more confident because you get thrown into different situations I have to get on with it. (Social Worker, Uganda)

I have learnt that I am a very strong person, I can do anything I put my mind to and it has also given me a lot more confidence as a student nurse, that I can carry forward to when I am qualified. (Nurse, Uganda)

Even just outside the placements spending a bit of time in a different country increases your confidence...not sure how I'll translate it into practice but I learnt a lot about being in difficult situations and how to handle them (laughs) and a lot about emotional intelligence and how to deal with conflict and things like that and how to manage like stress as well. (Occupational Therapist, Uganda)

When faced with the situations and experiences I did in Fort Portal, Uganda, I bloomed and I know for a fact that not only has it made me a better professional but that it has changed my life forever and will ultimately impact on my career and future planning of it. If I had the chance to go back and do it all over again I wouldn't change a thing. (Nurse, Uganda)

## Employability

Although a number of students expressed concern even at being asked about the impact of their placement on their future employability, perhaps sensing that this was unethical and sounded 'selfish' it was clear that students recognised the potential career-enhancing effects of the placement experience in terms of 'giving them the edge' or 'setting them apart'. Responses to the survey were overwhelmingly positive with 95% of students believing their placement was very beneficial for their future career and employability. This applied equally to students on observational placements. The following comments are typical:

It will show that I've got a determination expand my horizons and gain further experiences and take on challenges. (Nurse, India)

I never really thought 'this can go in my portfolio' and 'this can be good for jobs' but everyone's telling me, even on my last (UK) placement, 'that'll be really good for interviews and jobs'. (Physiotherapist, Uganda.

I think It puts me in a very strong position because in university they say all the time when it comes to job applications; have you done something that would make you stand out from the crowd...that automatically gives you a win in the interviews – you've got a really positive experience you can talk about all day – that makes you much more employable. (Nurse, Uganda)

It will give an edge, Not a lot of nurses do it so to do it as a student shows you can manage in a different setting. You can manage in scarce resources. You can work on your own, know your limits, you're resourceful. There's loads of indications to an employer that you can work under stressful situations with new encounters and work through it in a logical way to get the most out of it for your patient. So just by saying that you've done this to an employer shows you have all these qualities and shows that you will go that extra mile to go and make a difference and improve patient care. (Nurse, Uganda)

## SUMMARY

This chapter has summarised the findings of the survey and qualitative interviews to demonstrate the impact that educational placements have on student learning. The results show that the learning outcomes are profound and directly relevant to undergraduate curricular and NHS objectives. There was an overwhelming belief that the placements contributed to their future skills and employability. Unsurprisingly clinical skills learning was much more pronounced amongst students undertaking the EEP placement and experiencing hands-on clinical work under the direct supervision by Professional Volunteers and Ugandan health workers.

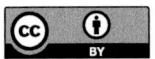

# CHAPTER 4

# Ethical Placements? Under What Conditions Can Educational Placements Support Sustainable Development?

## INTRODUCTION

Understanding the impact of human mobility on various forms of knowledge transfer and economic development has formed the subject of recent debate. Our sister book (Ackers and Ackers-Johnson 2016) is devoted to a wider discussion of the impact of the deployment of professional (i.e. qualified) volunteers on the Ugandan public health system. If there is a dearth of research on this topic and some scepticism about the impact of very highly skilled professionals undertaking extended stays in low resource settings, then it is fair to say that our understanding of the impact of short stay undergraduate electives is more or less non-existent. The literature on volunteer-tourism or 'voluntourism' has begun to raise uncomfortable questions but mainly within the frame of 'gap year' sojourns (Simpson 2004; Snee 2013). As we have noted, to the extent that there is any published research on electives it is almost exclusively focused on medical students (Coates 2006; Drain et al. 2007; Rominski et al. 2015). Some of this literature, whilst primarily focused on the (clinical) gains to the students themselves and the risks of what are quite often self-organised individual ventures, has hinted at the potential burden placed upon host locations (BMA 2009; Rominksi et al. 2015). As with all forms of 'volunteering' there is a presumption of benevolence, of altruism and inherent good or at least neutrality; of 'no harm'. But peppered within this fluffy

© The Author(s) 2017
A. Ahmed et al., *The Ethics of Educational Healthcare Placements in Low and Middle Income Countries*, DOI 10.1007/978-3-319-48363-4_4

celebratory glow is a thorny question; in a context when the UK is itself struggling to place, train and fund its own, why should we expect low resource settings to take responsibility for training its future health workforce?

Our role in the deployment of long-term volunteers has made us very aware of the need for careful recruitment and deployment within structured, supported and managed programmes if we are to avoid becoming part of the problem and undermining health systems. Indeed, this is an unfolding story of 'unintended consequences.' The EEP model builds on eight years' experience of managing volunteers in the context of the Ugandan *public* health system. Unlike other elective placement schemes run by private companies keen to profit from the burgeoning demand for international placements, the EEP model grew out of our Sustainable Volunteering Programme and is firmly situated within an active and evidence-based partnership-based engagement. The ethics and sustainability of our engagement has formed a key component of project design and evaluation.

Building on our previous (exploratory) experience of deploying medical students alongside professional volunteers we anticipated two key dimensions of (positive and sustainable) impact. In the first instance, we knew that professional volunteers working for long periods in highly stressful circumstances and often with reluctant learners and absent colleagues were often 'refreshed' and re-energised when UK students arrived. Secondly, having witnessed some very bad practice involving payments for supervision by small poorly organised income-generating electives programmes, we were aware of the pitfalls of cash inducements to local supervisors/ mentors. These payments typically failed to guarantee any supervision on the ground and contributed to systemic corruption. On the other hand, we witnessed the important contribution even quite small strategic investments could make to removing simple 'snags' that debilitate local health systems. Mdee and Emmott (2008) define the 'tension between operating a viable and commercially-sustainable enterprise and maximising social and development impacts' in the context of what they call 'pro poor tourism' (p. 191). Whilst we would distinguish undergraduate electives from gap year tourism the tension remains and lies at the heart of the EEP mission. The authors advocate the extension of a certification process based on Fair Trade Principles to kitemark organisations involved in volunteer deployment. Informed by these principles, the EEP project sought to design a model that reduced the risks of contributing to global inequality and corruption (through the commodification of placements) or systems dependency (on consumables provision for example) and enabled us to make systems enhancing investments.

Perhaps influenced by the somewhat negative experiences of 'free mover' medical electives[1] compounded by the voluntourism debates we had rather anticipated students aiding the knowledge brokering functions of professional volunteers and seriously underestimated the role that students themselves, when appropriately placed, can play in knowledge exchange processes. Our research has evidenced the important role that students can play in actively supporting mutual learning on-the-job in health facilities but also in conjunction with undergraduate teaching programmes. And, linked to this peer mentoring role, we have found that the student placements have had a significant motivational impact on health workers in the facilities they have been based in. Finally, as the project has developed we have sought to incentivise and invest in the skills and experiences of local health workers. This is not to suggest that Ugandan health workers lack the skills and experience to supervise UK students. But we are very aware of marked differences in role delineation, training and experience. With that in mind we have encouraged bi-lateral professional exchanges supporting Ugandan health workers to apply for fellowships to spend time in the UK. With the support of British Commonwealth Professional Fellowships, we have been able to bring a number of colleagues over from both the University and the Health District to experience British professional education and placement schemes and intensify the quality of relationships.

We have noted elsewhere the externality effects associated with 'gap-filling' and labour-substitution roles. Deploying volunteers in service delivery undermines local health systems (Ackers and Ackers-Johnson 2016). It is also associated with high levels of personal risk for volunteers. This is heightened in the case of students. As a result, all of our engagement is underpinned by the 'co-presence' principle reducing to a minimum the incidence of lone working. Our objectives are system-focused and we hope that such a focus will in the medium term improve the care of all patients and not just those whose lives we personally touch. Having said that we are acutely aware that very many patients have benefited on a daily basis from their encounters with

---

[1] Opengart uses the concept of 'free agent learners' in the context of boundaryless careers. In the past many medical students negotiated their own placements as individual 'pioneers'.

our students. Patients comment regularly on the care and compassion shown to them by British professionals and students and we are in absolutely no doubt that our students have saved the lives of mothers and babies and improved the quality of lives for many others.

Students were invited, in the survey, to comment on the impact they believed their placement had on the individuals, facilities, organisations and health system in the country within which they were placed. This is obviously a very broad and subjective question, and the students' responses may not be indicative of their actual impact. However, responses were very positive. Fifty-four percent of students believed they had a very positive impact, 34% a slightly positive impact and 9% no impact. Three percent of students were unsure, however no students believed their placement had a negative impact. The responses for students travelling to Uganda were generally more positive than those travelling to India, which is likely to be related to the fact that the India placement were observational only whereas the Uganda placements allowed for supervised hands-on practice as mentioned previously. Additionally, the health facilities and staffing in India were more advanced than those in Uganda which left more scope for students to try to make improvements in the Ugandan health facilities.

The remainder of this chapter assesses the ethics of placing students in Uganda because, as we have explained, the placements in India were organised on a very different basis. We had no prior engagement in India and the placements were organised by other parties in a private, not-for-profit health facility. The entire programme was managed by the Indian organisation which charged a fee for every student of £850.[2] It was clear from the start that these were observation only placements and students were prohibited from any involvement with patients or wards and they included a two-week non-clinical cultural exposure designed specifically for these and many other foreign students. The India placements did not set out to support local capacity-building or systems change and took place largely outside the Indian public health system. As such we do not regard these as falling within the model of 'Ethical Educational Placements'.

Chapter 2 emphasised the importance of systems change and capacity-building to all of our work in Uganda. This implies a focus on *public*

---

[2] This is usual practice with companies active in the electives market. What distinguishes this placement, however, is that there was no intermediary organisation in the UK taking a slice of the profits.

health systems and we have questioned the ethics and sustainability of investing in parallel service development in the private and not-for-profit sectors.[3] In this context, the chapter examines first the 'knowledge premium' associated with placements asking whether students play a role in the transfer and exchange of useful knowledge and skills. It then moves on to discuss the role that the EEPs have played in creating new opportunities for the kinds of active knowledge mobilisation necessary to bring about sustainable systems change.

## Supporting Professional Volunteer Engagement and Efficacy

Our decision to embark on the development of an ethical placements programme stemmed directly from our role in managing and evaluating the Sustainable Volunteering Program (SVP). The SVP deployed long-term highly skilled professional volunteers within the frame of the Ugandan Maternal and Newborn Hub to promote sustainable improvements in public health systems (as outlined in Chapter 2 and in Ackers and Ackers-Johnson 2016). Understanding the contribution that even these qualified volunteers can make towards sustainable system change has proved a real challenge. What we have learnt, over a period of many years, is that volunteer deployment and management is critical to mitigation of potential systems damage. Linked to this we have observed the mutual benefits of using long-term volunteers as anchors for short stays (Ackers 2015); short stays in the absence of continued project and personnel presence on the ground are rarely successful and can lapse into damaging forms of service delivery.[4] On the other hand, when there is continuity of clearly defined projects with on-going bridging relationships, short-term stays can be highly beneficial both in terms of harnessing critical skills and motivational impacts. And, having long term volunteers on the ground preparing for and creating the 'sticky branches' (Meyer 2003) that lubricate short stays enables short stay professionals to hit the

---

[3] Case Study 5 outlines work undertaken by a placement group focused on the development of a Public-Private-Partnership as outlined in the Ugandan Ministry of Health's Strategic Plan, 2012.

[4] It is continued presence over time rather than the length of individual stays that is of importance here.

ground running' and become effective knowledge brokers almost immediately. In this case, short stayers are most commonly very senior professionals unable to commit to longer periods away from work. However, we observed similar effects with short-stay medical electives; the Professional Volunteers were often excited to have students join them to support their own plans for audits or specific interventions. Motivation over the course of long-term placements often wanes in the face of on-going challenges (Gedde et al. 2011). At times, local health workers appear disinterested in training and long-term volunteers gain motivation from having knowledge-hungry UK students on the wards as the following volunteer suggests:

> They (group of nursing students) have been some of the best students I've ever supervised. They were always on time, keen to learn and got straight on with whatever needed to be done that day . . . It removes some of the stress having more people around to help out. (PV, Uganda)

The SVP came to an abrupt end, as with many development interventions, when our knowledge of how to mobilise and optimally place volunteers was at its peak. This is an on-going problem with Aid with many projects; jumping between funded programmes and defining themselves according to the demands of funders rather than the evidence-base and longer term strategic but iterative objectives. We realised that if we were able to mobilise an effective placement programme and generate an overhead that could fund the placement of long-term volunteers, we could achieve the kind of symbiotic sustainability capable of achieving incremental evidence-based systems impact.

Chapter 3 has discussed the benefits of long term volunteers to student support and learning. Our concern in this chapter is to explain how the model as a whole underwrites the deployment of long-term volunteers (as an outcome for host institutions and systems). It could be argued that investing in mobile expertise from the UK (in the form of professional volunteers) is in itself an example of neo-colonialism. Why not utilise local expertise to fulfil the supervisory role? Sadly, our experience of managing PVs in Uganda has exposed the fundamental weaknesses of human resource management systems in the Ugandan public health system. Elsewhere, we have argued that the failure to implement effective human resource management processes to counter endemic absenteeism and poor time-keeping lies at the heart of maternal morbidity and mortality (Ackers et al. 2016). Absenteeism is a major problem in Uganda and many staff either fail to come to work at all or, when they do, tend to show very poor attitudes towards time-keeping. This problem is common to many low resource settings where systems of accountability are not in place and creates a specific challenge for the organisation of undergraduate placements. This is one of the key reasons why professional volunteers are so important to minimise the risks associated with lone working and ensure effective supervision in often extremely stressful circumstances. Asked whether the impact of the EEP would be the same without the presence of professional volunteers, a lecturer at Mountains of the Moon University replied:

> If you don't they (the UK students) won't get supervised – it would be dangerous to do that.

In a far more complex process, the deployment of professional volunteers in turn supports the development of training clusters that have a centrifugal effect in drawing in local health workers and students. Put more metaphorically; the professional volunteers can be characterised as the eyes of creative (and disruptive) knowledge mobilisation storms. But building and sustaining clusters is labour intensive. It requires organisation, planning, active bi-lateral communication and on-the-ground co-presence. These clusters and the benefits accruing from them cannot be achieved by simply posting large volumes of students in low resource settings and paying a cash premium. The following respondent (a member of staff at the local university) responds to the question, 'Could we have MMU and our students working alongside on placement?'

> Yes, that would be great so long as we don't have too many there at once – it depends a bit on the timing and numbers. It would be good if we communicated a bit better and tried to line it up a bit more.

As we have noted above, during the SVP it was rare to see anything other than medical students on electives. The opportunity to deploy much wider cadres of students has contributed significantly to this process creating opportunities for multi-disciplinary exchanges supporting the work of professional volunteers in a more holistic way. An example of this can be seen in the deployment of child nursing students into the neonatal units linked to maternal facilities. This has provided critical support to our obstetric and midwifery volunteers attempting to care for mothers and babies from pregnancy until they are able to go home. It provided opportunities for students to 'spoke out' to witness birthing processes and immediate neonatal care, and then follow this through to the neonatal unit. In effect, it enables the volunteers to be in two places at once but always at hand if the students need support. In the process the UK nurses are able to work alongside, and share their skills and experience with, local staff and students. In a similar vein, students have been able to be actively involved in ante-natal or baby clinics, in laboratory-based testing of patients or in record keeping and management, all of which support the complex interventions of long-term volunteers. It is clear from our research that undergraduate students play an active role in augmenting the knowledge brokerage function of long-term volunteers.

## Students as Knowledge Brokers

Having conceptualised UK professional volunteers as knowledge brokers (Ackers and Ackers-Johnson 2016) we are nevertheless aware of some tension between the needs and ability to exercise long-term mobility on the part of UK professionals, on the one hand, and the expressed needs of host institutions for the most senior clinicians. Our experience of the volunteers has challenged received wisdom on the part of UK professional bodies (such as the Royal Colleges), volunteer deployment agencies (such as VSO) and Ugandan hosts that only very senior clinicians are suitable and able to make a serious contribution. Indeed, some of the most effective volunteers have been more junior doctors willing to engage in some of the more mundane back-to-basics systems repair work. We were not expecting students, caricatured in roles as learners (inert sponges) rather than 'teachers' to assume the role of knowledge brokers. Our research indicates quite the opposite; that the students we have selected, in the positions we have placed them and with the support in place, have played very active and meaningful knowledge brokerage roles. Many interventions (such as triage, infection control or medical records audit for example) benefit from having more human resource to assist. The emphasis on 'back-to-basics' or 'neglected processes'[5] in global health lends itself well to less experienced cadres especially when they are carefully

---

[5] The concept of 'neglected processes' was utilised within the frame of the Ugandan Maternal and Newborn Hub interventions at the suggestion of Dr Simon Mardel.

supervised and managed. Mardel, a leading expert of ebola-preparedness work, describes the key global health challenges as follows:

> The greatest currently achievable gains in global healthcare appear dependent on solving the currently 'neglected' processes in organisation and delivery of health care and health education. These deficits, aimed at disease prevention, early diagnosis, self-care, low cost intervention, early recognition of severity, appropriate and safe use of existing resources are not sufficiently covered by existing specialties, or their redress requires unprecedented collaboration.[6]

We have reproduced Mardel's '7 pillars' in Fig. 4.1 to illustrate the potential contribution that undergraduate students can make to global health. Improving these basic processes such as patient monitoring, record keeping, IPC and access to information are precisely the areas where students have the knowledge and skills to engage effectively with local health workers and health systems in critical public and preventive health roles. This explains why, in many respects, we believe that knowledge mobilisation clusters combining undergraduate students with UK midwifery, nursing and AHP volunteers (and their Ugandan peers) deliver optimal impact.

One of the contexts within which this knowledge brokerage role has occurred most proactively has been through their engagement with Ugandan students. We had anticipated and planned to 'buddy' the students with our partner University (Mountains of the Moon) and this has created opportunities for more formal mutual learning encounters; similar to the buddy system employed in India. Many of the students have taken advantage of this opportunity and planned joint workshops and seminars with their student peers at MMU and Makerere University. One of the local supervisors made the following comment on peer learning showing its motivational impact on them as trainers and the students involved:

> It was a great opportunity to sit together and analyse; 'what do you study that we don't study and what do we study that you don't study' so it was a great opportunity for all the students. And to us, the trainers, it was very interesting to know how students from the UK think and how they look at things because that guides us on what we can also tell our students. You

---

[6] Cited at http://www.nhsevents.org/img/events/213/Dr%20Simon%20Mardell.pdf

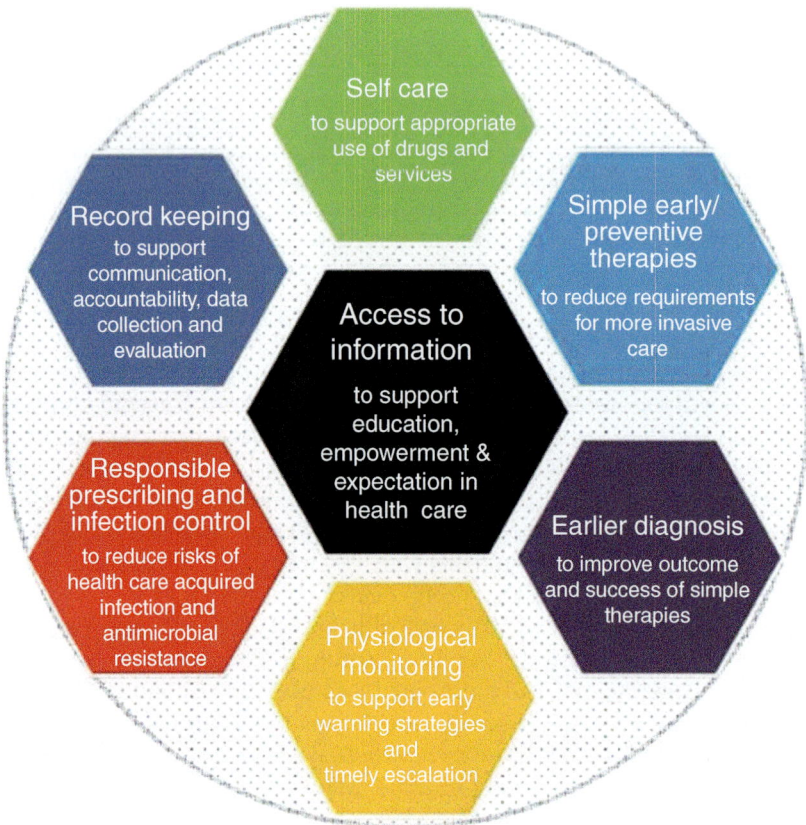

**Fig. 4.1**  The seven pillars of neglect in global health. *Source*: Acknowledgement to come

know we are always limited with some few things and sometimes we pick-up the perception of maybe we cannot get this far but with the interaction we had with them we realised that yes if we pick up that kind of thinking and try to initiate it into our students then we'll have the best out of this program.

This programme is continuing to evolve and we are currently hosting this respondent in the UK on a 5-month Commonwealth Professional Fellowship focused on prosthetics and robotics. The Fellowship is designed to build relationships for future undergraduate placements but also to support capacity-building in Uganda in the development of prosthetics. This in turn represents an immediate response to a very tragic case of domestic violence (Case Study 1):

## CASE STUDY 1: HOLISTIC RESPONSES TO DOMESTIC VIOLENCE

In June 2016, a young mother from a very isolated rural area was brutally attacked by her partner who hacked off both of her hands and caused serious injury to her face including the loss of an ear and an eye. Ninsiima is a peasant farmer with two small children and was thirty-six weeks pregnant at the time of the attack. She was cared for, from an obstetric perspective, by a K4C professional volunteer and gave birth safely. Students on the EEP placements then supported her to care for her baby in the newly set up neo-natal unit prior to her return home. At this point a group of young pioneering engineers that had been trained by the University of Salford/K4C biomedical engineering project[7] under the leadership of Dr Ssekitoleko responded to the situation. One of these engineers (Mr Senabulya) became involved in assessing the possibility of building prosthetic hands for Ninsiima. This lead to a successful application for funding to the British Commonwealth Fellowship programme, enabling Mr Senabulya to come to Salford University for five months to work with colleagues in robotics and prosthetics. The objective of this fellowship is to build capacity in Uganda in the production of prosthetics for low resource settings, assess the possibility of building two hands for Ninsiima whilst also working alongside the UK placement team to build on our successful prosthetics and orthotics placements. One of the EEP students placed in this environment explains her experience:

> The first two weeks were based in the largest referral hospital in Uganda. We were looking at things like fractures, spinal injuries and club foot. We were helping out as much as we could and seeing patients on a daily basis and looking at the challenges they faced and trying to sort out solutions to make it easier for them by reducing the cost of things and the kind of materials they needed because the lack of resources was one of the main problems over there. The second two weeks we were with the students from the orthopaedic medical school, essentially it is just the same course as we are doing. They

[7] This project is funded by the Tropical Health and Education Trust. For details see http://www.salford.ac.uk/research/care/research-groups/knowledge-and-place

were doing prosthetics, dealing with wheelchairs and crutches. We were seeing what we could learn from them and teach them what we have learned here. (Prosthetics & Orthotics, Uganda)

EEP students have also provided considerable support to our PVs involved in the assessment of the MMU midwifery degree students in OSCI-type clinical scenarios.[8] All of the people involved in these have found them immensely valuable. One of the MMU lecturers expresses her views about the students' contribution:

*Interviewer:*   "Do you feel the students make an active contribution to Uganda – do they have skills to give or are they too junior?"

*MMU Lecturer:*   "I have met a few groups who have done some teaching with our students then on Saturday [the volunteer] had them come and help with a mock OSCI with the MMU students and I observed that. It's also helpful to our students in lectures – they see a student with a different capacity – with more knowledge and skills.

*Interviewer:*   "So you feel the UK students have more knowledge and skills than MMU students?"

*MMU Lecturer:*   "Probably like with the clinical examinations [the volunteer] is using the UK students for the actual exam; they can read an exam question and act appropriately; they know the practical side. The MMU students don't. Observing the UK students on the wards in comparison to other nursing schools in Fort Portal who send students with zero clinical skills; your students are teaching these Ugandan students on the wards. Our MMU midwives are pretty experienced but many of the other students in Fort Portal are not. The [EEP students'] clinical practice is different and at a higher standard than here so they are model clinicians in a student role. [LTV] has commented that she really thinks they add a lot to the general student population who come to the hospital for clinical placements. And with the SVP volunteers mentoring your students there is a wealth of knowledge – a real cluster which is of real benefit to the local students.

---

[8] An 'objective structured clinical examination' (OSCE) is a modern type of 'hands-on' examination often used in health sciences designed to test clinical skill performance and competence. (https://en.wikipedia.org/wiki/Objective_structured_clinical_examination)

EEP students have also been actively engaged in CPD-style training in health facilities and the community. Nursing and paramedic EEP students developed bespoke first aid training programmes for cadres of staff who have never had the opportunity for training; most notably these included all the local ambulance drivers and a group of potential paramedics. Wherever possible, we support opportunities for training interventions involving the students. As a project, we have a firm policy on cash per diems (we never pay them) and we endeavour to hold the training as close as possible and where we can within the clinical environment to reduce time out of work (see Ackers and Ackers-Johnson 2016). What we had perhaps underestimated was the very important knowledge brokerage role that EEP students played in relation to other (Ugandan) students and health workers. Here the benefits were mutual with active exchanges of skills and experience taking place. In the case of many Ugandan students,[9] the more advanced knowledge/experience of the UK students (most of whom are at the end of their second year and/or mature students) meant that the UK students filled the roles of the usually absent local supervisors.

We noted above the involvement of UK students in paramedic training to ambulance drivers and nurses. At first we had some anxiety about placing students from Allied Health Professions that do not (yet) exist in Ugandan public services. These concerned, in particular, paramedics and podiatrists. It proved difficult to explain to many Ugandan health workers what a podiatrist was. However, we were able to place them in a club foot and diabetic clinic in a local hospital and this precipitated a strong demand for more such students on the part of the hospital and the expression of interest in further developing work on diabetic foot ulcers (a speciality of some of the Salford tutors). Similarly, discussions with the District Health Officer about the placement of paramedics raised the possibility of working towards a policy of requiring a local health worker to accompany patients on ambulance journeys alongside the drivers (who currently travel

---

[9] We are referring here to the large numbers of new entrants into certificate and diploma level nursing studying at colleges in Fort Portal and not to the Diploma qualified experienced midwives on the MMU degree.

unaccompanied). How far ideas such as they progress remains to be seen; what we can say with some certainty is that the placement of students and exposure to the diverse professions has had an impact in terms of policy transfer. As a project, we make careful decisions about whether and how to invest in these project ideas that arise during placements in a very cautious and iterative fashion.

In the next case the manager of one of our partner organisations, an experienced British physiotherapist, explains how she felt the students contributed to her own reflective practice and to the mentoring of Ugandan staff within the organisation:

> It was really good for us to learn from them because they kept on asking why we do things – it makes you as a clinician think about what you are doing more. Instead of just doing what I do I have to explain it and think about it. It's what Ugandan students don't do. They're anxious about questioning. Our physios here enjoy learning from the UK students. They bring the latest research; local staff don't have the same level of education.

The point about local staff reflects in many ways the nascence of some of these allied health professions in low resource settings such as Uganda. It is not a comment about the innate abilities of local staff or students but the fact that most of them will be qualified at certificate or diploma level. In comparison, many of the UK physiotherapy students already held a first degree. The respondent (above) goes on to make a point about length of stay in the placement setting suggesting that from the perspective of her investment and the benefits of the local organisation students are best placed in one location for most of the time:

> We try to do a lot of teaching and set objectives for each student. Throughout their first week we looked at their strengths and weaknesses, and say ok let's work on your weaknesses while you are here! So, it's very individualised and that's what we can do when somebody is here for 3 weeks, but not when somebody is only here for 2 days. And also, you don't want to put so much time and effort in, I just don't have the same interest because in 2 days they're not going to learn that much from me, as opposed to three weeks, they have a huge amount of things they can learn, we can sit down and do teaching sessions and discuss cases. But

I'm not going to do that with somebody who's only here for 2 days, because it's a lot of time and effort on my part and they don't get the same out of it. It's not fair on the parents, that you constantly have a new person working on their child.

Another Ugandan supervisor makes a similar comment suggesting he would prefer stays of two months:

| | |
|---|---|
| *Interviewer:* | *"Are students too junior (not skilled enough) to be of use to Uganda – are they more of a burden than a benefit?* |
| *Ugandan Supervisor:* | *"No, I wouldn't call it a burden because learning is both sides; some things we learn from them so it is experience sharing. It isn't a burden the only challenge is the time they spend – if it is not too much time then the orientation ends when their period here is ending. In one month they get used to everything and then the second month they could perform but we do benefit".* |

This is an interesting issue which reflects some creative tension between the wishes of students, in some cases, to experience a breadth of settings and exposures. The EEP placement team have tried to balance these needs and explain to the students the risks of volunteer tourism and voyeurism and the importance to their learning and impacts of relationship-building. Rominksi et al refer to this as a necessary process of 'expectation management' (2015: 3). On the other hand, some students found their placements extremely demanding. This very much depended on the context rather than the student in question. Placements on a very busy neonatal unit whilst very interesting and rewarding (and the envy of many EEP students) are exhausting. In this situation one of the students felt that a day a week in another setting was helpful:

It was nice to have one day a week to do something that gave relief and fun. Something through which you could understand the community a bit more. Like the health clinic, that was good. (Midwife, Uganda)

The compromise we have developed is to give students a flexible half day on a Friday to enable them to negotiate visits to other settings whilst keeping them firmly anchored in their primary location. This process in itself forms a critical part of student learning about global health.

## THE 'FAIR TRADE PREMIUM': LOCAL INVESTMENT WITHOUT FOSTERING CORRUPTION

One of the most obvious ways to compensate or reimburse hosts in low resource settings for the work they do in supervising and mentoring UK students is via direct cash payments and, arguably, this is the mechanism that extends optimal autonomy to partners in the host setting enabling them to identify their own investment objectives. Many for-profit placement providers make cash payments directly into organisations (hospitals) as is the case in the Makerere/Mulago International Electives Programme or, often more informally, to local in-charges or senior health staff on the wards. In our experience neither of these approaches avoids the pitfalls associated with endemic corruption especially in the public sector or puts systems in place to guarantee supervision. Student placements become commodified and students are treated as 'cash cows' creating opportunities for personal gain. [10]

We have witnessed the 'institutional' approach in the National Referral Hospital where student placements have become an element of income generation, resulting not so much in a lack of supervision (in this incidence) but more in a kind of 'herding' of large volumes of students through wards in an almost voyeuristic enterprise. This process creates a serious burden for overwhelmed local staff and ward managers working in very congested facilities with few staff. One manager of a large maternity facility in Kampala told us that she felt that most of her time was spent supervising students. She was quick to point out that many of these were bussed into the hospital from local nursing and midwifery schools in large and unpredictable numbers but this was compounded by groups of visiting students from overseas. In addition to distracting local staff this herding process compounds physical congestion and existing problems of patient privacy, confidentiality and infection prevention control.

During the SVP, we also identified cases where small UK charities have engaged in student recruitment to aid their fund raising and organised, in

---

[10] Placements in the UK are remunerated on an inter-institutional basis but systems are in place to ensure accountability and supervision.

good faith, at a distance cash payments to local clinical leaders. We have witnessed directly these payments being taken on a personal basis by senior (and mostly absent) managers with no funds trickling down to benefit the staff working on the ground. This creates tensions, jealousies and, most critically, results in lone working. We have discussed in some detail in our sister volume (Ackers and Ackers-Johnson 2016) issues around the commodification of training in Uganda and do not have space to rehearse these issues here. What is absolutely clear from all perspectives is that student placements have been recognised as a lucrative marketable commodity by both sending[11] and receiving organisations resulting in some quite unethical outcomes.

In order to avoid these risks whilst also recognising the importance of some compensatory function we have adopted a 'Fair Trade Premium' approach. The previous section has evidenced the complexity of multilateral knowledge exchange processes associated with EEPs. Transferring knowledge in itself will fail to precipitate systems change in Ugandan public health facilities as knowledge mobilisation requires that health workers not only have knowledge but are also motivated to use that knowledge and have access to a basic modicum, of resource to facilitate behaviour change.[12] In this context the 'Fair Trade Premium' is not simply compensatory; it represents a critical investment in knowledge mobilisation processes.

In practice this has involved setting aside £150 from each placement to support critical local investments that facilitate effective placements and systems improvement. The Premium takes the form of negotiated 'in-kind' investments: we never pay cash. Working with well-established local partners we identify 'snagging' problems that a small, immediate investment could overcome. Examples include the provision of a placenta pit in a facility where the lack of such a resource was the main factor preventing patient admissions. No amount of training or knowledge transfer could have got this maternity facility functioning if there was no way of disposing of placentas. We have also repaired or installed sinks as a precursor to hand hygiene training to support our infection

---

[11] It is certainly true to say that the clamouring gap year companies are making the biggest financial gains here not the hosting organisations.

[12] These relationships are discussed in more detail in Ackers and Ackers-Johnson (2016) (Chapter 4).

prevention control interventions whilst also reducing risks for students. In other cases, we have constructed patient waiting areas to enable patients to wait under cover for out-patient treatment rather than congesting corridors. This also then created a visible space for students to set up a triage area and 'role model' the taking of basic observations and basic record-keeping. We have also undertaken some improvements to accommodation to enable doctors to remain on site during their duties; there was a property but it had fallen into some disrepair and needed some basic re-wiring and plumbing to connect water and power. Our intervention here was aimed at improving the medical presence to ensure 24/7 cover as audit work had shown that the lack of medical presence was responsible for high levels of inappropriate referrals (and maternal and neonatal deaths). We also know that having doctors on site at all times created a better learning environment for our students. Other 'investments' included support to the university to provide transport for their own students (an on-going problem in Uganda) which would also in theory benefit the placement students and urgent repairs to an ambulance. We had some reservations about this last investment as we do not wish to get involved in covering any routine running costs or consumables. However, at the time none of the five ambulances were on the road and we wanted to utilise the opportunity of having three UK paramedic students to encourage the development of basic first-aid training to ambulance drivers and, more symbolically, to push policy makers to begin to consider the possibility of paramedic support to ambulance drivers. In practice, we were right to have such reservations as the ambulance was out of service again a month later. We have also purchased books for the university library and supported the costs of a mobile HIV/cancer screening/family planning clinic.[13]

The following section discusses these 'investments' in more detail to illustrate their knowledge mobilisation function. The following Ugandan ward manager describes her appreciation of the investments the EEP has made in the Regional Referral Hospital (RRH), the facility in which she was based:

---

[13] See Case Study 4 below.

| | |
|---|---|
| *Interviewer:* | *"Do you think your practice has changed in any way as a result of the students being here?"* |
| *Ward Manager (RRH):* | *"Maybe hand hygiene, when they gave us the hand washing gel. They gave us books; we can consult from those books. We have about four textbooks on occupational therapy and mental health; it is helping us as we didn't have any at all"* |

This quote illustrates the value of these 'in-kind' contributions not as isolated donations but as part of active programs of intervention on the ground. The hand gel referred to by the respondent was manufactured as part of an ongoing THET-funded project on Infection Prevention Control.[14]

## CASE STUDY 2: REDUCING MATERNAL MORTALITY THROUGH INFECTION PREVENTION CONTROL

The ground work for this intervention commenced several years earlier as part of the SVP project in response to concerns about the lack of Ebola preparedness in Uganda. In the first instance, an SVP volunteer began local production of alcohol hand rub in a public facility in Kampala. This worked extremely well. However, when the project funding stopped, so did production of the gel despite very minimal production costs and apparent high-level stakeholder support.

K4C decided to repeat this process but with stronger sustainability elements built in including production of an accredited product (registered with the Uganda National Bureau of Standards) with potential for sales into the private sector (as a social enterprise). Having this on-going project in Kabarole provided exciting opportunities for student engagement in all aspects of the work. UK students working alongside local university (MMU) students have played an active role in all stages of this intervention including the Infrastructure Audit (a WHO instrument designed to assess the presence of sinks; running water, soap etc.); active hand hygiene training some of which was student-lead; the manufacture and marketing of the product and audit using a modified WHO Hand Hygiene Compliance Tool. This kind of managed intervention has quite a different impact to simply giving local staff bottles of hand gel.

---

[14] www.knowledge4change.org.uk/

One of the EEP students played a particularly important role in this project. He applied for a placement as a mature social work student. He had previously worked for over ten years in a pharmaceutical company (Apollo Scientific Research, Manchester)[15] and began to apply his skills and knowledge in this area many months prior to deployment raising funding for infrastructural investments and working with his previous employer to provide over 2000 plastic bottles to help the hand gel production process. Invited to reflect on his impact on the ground he replied:

> It is a case now of following it through because it is a long term project and I'm happy with that. I'm speaking to [local staff and UK Company] about it on a regular basis and I am happy to stay involved. Some things are worth putting energy into and this is one of them. I think seeds were sown with the hand gel.

Student placements have provided very valuable support to this intervention which has in return created a real-life experience of IPC interventions for the students. This student, who is now doing a doctorate at another university, is continuing to support the work in Uganda. His interview underlines the importance of project continuity to effective placements but also to local health systems. It also reminds us that many undergraduate students have extensive life experience and skills accrued prior to their current degree. Indeed, many of the EEP students had prior degrees and most of them have extensive work experience.

The Ugandan biomedical engineer who acted as the local supervisor of the prosthetic and orthotic EEP students commented on the value he and his University gained from the investments made in purchasing local materials for the EEP students to use in the manufacture of prosthetics for local patients. These also benefitted their Ugandan student peers and of course the patients they treated. At his request we also purchased a projector to help in the delivery of training during the placements and beyond:

> We really benefited a lot because the school of orthopaedic medicine got materials that it had not gotten before and the school of orthopaedic technology also got materials plus the projector that went to the school of orthopaedic medicine. These things they needed but they could not get

---

[15] Apollo Scientific Research are now underwriting the costs of providing bottles and labels for the gel.

them from the administration because of the limited funds so when this project came in we told them we should make sure that the money should support the actual school that is involved. It's not going to the entire institution and that really so much benefited us.

This case illustrates the contribution that carefully managed investments can make in a much-grounded manner – which top-down Aid has so patently failed to achieve. They are small things that are of immediate benefit to the placement students themselves who in this case presented their work every week using the projector. There are very many cases in Uganda of students taking vocational courses who lack the raw materials to undertake practical work. We have witnessed this through our sister construction project (OBAAT)[16] where students lack access to protective clothing (including boots) basic equipment and raw materials such as cement or sand to enable them to actually practice building work.

Once the partners begin to recognise the value of these contributions and the fact that *no cash transfers will ever take place* the project began to settle. Indeed, we are rarely now asked for cash unless students are placed in the larger hospitals where there is an existing culture of such payments from local as well as international institutions. Interestingly, even when local colleges are charged a fee for placements we are not asked to follow suit. We believe that this reflects two things: firstly, that the UK students are often more highly trained and able to contribute more immediately than their Ugandan peers (or at least those cohorts who come straight from school). And, secondly, linked to that, the presence of the professional volunteers who in effect supervise/mentor their own staff plus the Ugandan students are in effect making their own non-pecuniary contribution. It is not so much that we are passing the responsibility for student supervision onto already hard pressed Ugandan staff: rather that, as a project, we are contributing to multi-disciplinary training and mentoring clusters.

Context is all important and in the environment within which the students are placed in Uganda we believe this is an effective, ethical and sustainable way of organising student placements. Notwithstanding the care taken to prevent the cash nexus fostering corruption and jealousy, we have had several experiences of Ugandan health workers trying to

---

[16] http://www.vmminternational.org/one-brick-at-a-time-obaat/

exhort cash from students. In one case a student (who incidentally came herself from Kenya and was black) was immediately pressurised to take bribes from patients as the doctor clearly did on a daily basis. He advised her that she would not survive long in Kenya if she did not engage in this practice (assuming she was going to be working in Kenya). In this case, despite talking to the doctor concerned, we decided to move the student to another location. In another and more common case, staff asked students to purchase drugs ostensibly to treat sick patients. We are aware that whilst this may be legitimate in some cases, this is also a mechanism to fund drugs for sale or for use in their private practices. On that basis, the project has adopted a firm stance on all donations urging students to report any such requests and resist the temptation to donate even small items, such as sweets and toys as this in itself distorts the objectives of the placements and the wider project and generates unintended consequences.

## From 'Ninja Medicine' to 'Neglected Processes'

We talked above about the unintended consequences of service delivery and gap-filling. This is a major risk with professional volunteers and especially more senior cadres many of whom are attracted by the lure of 'ninja medicine'.[17] Interestingly it has been less of a challenge with students perhaps because the students themselves respect the fact that they are primarily there to learn and more acutely aware of the risks of lone working. We have found this to be particularly the case with nursing, midwifery and allied health students who tend to show a higher level of humility, and perhaps a little less confidence (hubris) than medical students. The most pressing need in the Ugandan public health system is to attend to 'neglected processes' and get the basics right; if the basics could be improved we would be far less likely to see the kinds of emergencies that congest the main hospitals. EEP students played a very important role in supporting the back-to-basics orientation. In this capacity, they are supporting and working alongside local staff in critical role modelling

[17] This is a phrase used by a junior doctor in the SVP excited by the opportunities to save lives in emergency situations on a daily basis in the National Referral Hospital.

positions and, in the process, relieving the burden on them as the following Ugandan midwife explains:

> When a patient comes it is much quicker because everything is done on time when they are here. All the observations are done before we even touch the mother and the mothers do appreciate by the way. They come and tell us because they can't communicate with the students because of the language problem so they tell us. They say where did you get these doctors and nurses I wish you could keep bringing them because they are helping us a lot spending a lot of time on the mother so we wait less hours. Even in the late hours if we get a case they will come and help us. They ask questions when they don't understand because some of them are nurses and they also want to learn. For us here it is fantastic I may say.
> [Does it make more work for you?]
> No it is very easy it makes our work simpler. They were even very happy helping us with deliveries.

Involving students in preventive public health roles such as these can play a very important role in improving patient management, reducing congestion in overwhelmed referral hospitals and preventing damaging delays. Having said, that unless the students are placed in an environment of planned and active partnership founded on trust relationships these outcomes may not be realised. The respondent in the case above is a midwife in a health centre that we have been actively building links with for some years. Case Study 3 provides some background:

## CASE STUDY 3: SUSTAINABLE CAPACITY-BUILDING AT KAGOTE HEALTH CENTRE, KABAROLE DISTRICT

The midwife in the case above is based at Kagote Health Centre III, a midwifery-led unit based in Kabarole District. The first project visit to Kagote Health Centre took place in May, 2014. At this time the facility had not delivered a mother for 16 years and the maternity unit was closed. In June 2014 K4C organised a visit involving four self-funded students. Working alongside an SVP midwife volunteer and the wider project team the facility was opened for business within a month. We have continued to support this location through the deployment of professional volunteers and it became the first 'training site' for undergraduate placements.

A combination of our Fair-Trade contributions, working in close partner-ship with OBAAT, resulted in the relocation of the laboratory, the con-struction of two patient waiting areas; the refurbishment and extension of the delivery and post-natal wards and the relocation and refurbishment of the Out Patients Department. We have also been awarded Commonwealth Professional Fellowships for three of the five midwives based in Kagote to undertake further midwifery training at Salford University. This Health Centre was recently pronounced by the District Health Officer to be a model for Kabarole District. We are now using this site as a training site placement for MMU midwifery students who are supervised by both the local midwives and the SVP volunteers. The benefits for patients of this intervention can be seen in the graph shown in Fig. 4.2 produced during an audit undertaken by a recent placement trainee (in this case a Graduate Trainee from the Central Manchester Foundation Trust):

The very positive experience referred to above, and echoed by all mid-wives we interviewed, was not always shared by other cadres and in other contexts where our engagement as a project was less well-established or supported by long-term volunteers. We noted above the problems of motivation in the Ugandan public health workforce. The impact of poor motivation and a local culture[18] of absenteeism extends beyond the stu-dent's own learning to seriously reduce the potential impact of their presence. An on-going problem we face in placing students in Ugandan public health facilities is that we can only rarely rely on local staff to be present with any predictability or reliability. We are using the word 'cul-ture' here to refer not in an essentialist way to Ugandan ethnicities but

---

[18] We are using the word 'culture' here to refer not in an essentialist way to Ugandan ethnicities but rather to specific occupational sub-cultures within the public health sector. Corruption and absenteeism are a case in point. Interestingly we have found that absenteeism and poor time-keeping is less of a problem in midwifery in comparison to nursing, however, perhaps due to the fact that there is much greater pressure on midwives to be present on a 24/7 service. Many are not and many facilities operate a very limited week-day only service bit where this does take place mothers vote with their feet and either fail to access services at all or go directly to higher level referral facilities. On the whole midwives are far more likely to be present over the working day and to undertake night shifts than nursing staff working in Out Patient Departments who typically leave by 1 pm to engage in other forms of employment and supplement subsistence wages.

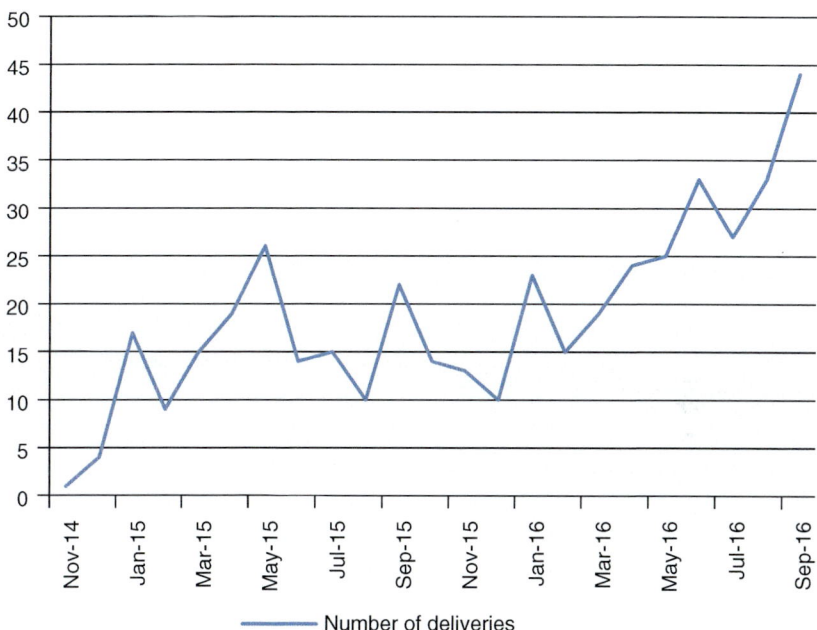

**Fig. 4.2** Deliveries at Kagote health centre, Kabarole district. *Source*: Created by the authors based on data collected on site by an EEP Placement Trainee, working alongside local midwives

rather to specific occupational sub-cultures within the public health sector. Corruption and absenteeism are a case in point. Interestingly we have found that absenteeism and poor time-keeping is less of a problem in midwifery in comparison to nursing, however, perhaps due to the fact that there is much greater pressure on midwives to be present on a 24/7 service. Many are not and many facilities operate a very limited week-day only service bit where this does take place mothers vote with their feet and either fail to access services at all or go directly to higher level referral facilities. On the whole midwives are far more likely to be present over the working day and to undertake night shifts than nursing staff working in Out Patient Departments who typically leave by 1 pm to engage in other forms of employment and supplement subsistence wages.

At most health centres there is strong pressure on nursing staff to 'clear the lines' (of patients) before 1 pm. This encourages staff to rush and is a major factor explaining the lack of effective patient monitoring and triage. In this environment, local staff may find having students around doing monitoring and triage effectively actually slows them down and this can generate some resentment to the presence of both students and professional volunteers. Patients are fully aware of this culture. As a result, many facilities (and potential placement locations) empty after 1 pm. This situation is reflected in the following responses:

> She only worked from 9 until 1 and then she'd go home. To begin with I would stay until one and then she sends me home. (Occupational Therapist, Uganda)
> I think they're just lazy because it always finishes by lunchtime: they can arrive late, see their patients quickly and then go home for lunch and then not turn up for the rest of the day. (Podiatrist, Uganda)

Where projects are actively engaged on the ground and where professional volunteers are in place this is much easier to predict and manage but nevertheless remains a major challenge for placement managers. An obvious response to this tension for placement managers is to place students in private and mission (not-for profit) facilities where occupational cultures (and human resource management) is quite different and supports a full working day and potentially more effective supervision. Our (ethical) commitment to health systems change could not support this approach and students would gain very little exposure to the challenges facing health systems in low resource settings if we took the easy option. Our commitment to co-presence further exacerbates this problem and the challenge of achieving active clinical engagement across the working day. If we allowed professional volunteers to engage in service delivery roles in the absence of local staff we could provide the supervision necessary to enable students to engage in clinical work. We have witnessed this type of situation on many occasions during visits to health centres. It is not at all unusual to see a quite junior overseas volunteer working with a small group of foreign students (often from different countries) on their own in a health facility. We would not regard this type of activity as either safe or ethically acceptable encouraging as it does systems damaging practices of absenteeism and moonlighting (Ackers et al. 2016).

The student in the following case explains how this situation affected his placement and the impacts associated with it. He experienced absenteeism in the hospital but also when the students had agreed to organise First Aid training for local ambulance staff and MMU students. Fortunately, he reflected on this as part of his own learning:

> There was a lot of absenteeism from Ugandan staff – some days I'd be going to the operating theatres and you would be all ready to go but no staff there so theatre would be cancelled. This obviously affects your entire day. With the staff absenteeism, that could affect our time because we could have prepared way in advance to go to do something and people don't turn up and then it is cancelled so that can be frustrating. It appears that even if they didn't come to work, they would still get paid, and then they questioned why there was such an issue with attendance. It's more about the situation in Uganda as opposed to us, but I don't know how we could possibly get it changed as it is outside our control. It was just interesting to see. (Adult Nurse, Uganda)

In another case the student suggested that local staff tried to 'put them out of their way'; they also observed that when the UK obstetrician volunteer was around local staff took the opportunity not to come to work (something we try hard to prevent):

> I think they just wanted us out of the way, so they put us in a room triaging, but they didn't listen to anything we said. When [professional volunteer] came the doctors stopped turning up because she was there to do the work. (Adult Nurse, Uganda)

In another context, students noted that when the Project Managers were around staff behaved quite differently towards them:

> It was really laid back. Have you heard that if it's raining people don't go to work they just stay indoors? The impression that we got is that when yourself and [X] go over, it's like the CQC (Care Quality Commission) coming to the hospitals over here, so there were certain staff that weren't very friendly towards us, or motivated. But when [X] was here she was saying that they were absolutely lovely they did everything but we had seen a completely different side of that. (Nurse, Uganda)

As a project, we learnt that placing some cadres of students presented more challenges than others and mental health was a case in point. In the first instance, we placed these students in the Mental Health Unit at the regional referral hospital aware that there was no community mental health in the Ugandan public system. This placement proved a serious challenge as the demands on language were much higher (most patients not speaking English and language being a much more important component of diagnosis and treatment). The Unit also managed the most serious cases with very few staff. This facility also completed its work around lunchtime each day and our interview with a local health worker expressed concerns at the lack of opportunity for active student engagement and the pressure this put on her:

> There are days here where I don't know what to do with these students when I am not busy and you have to make them busy so that was a very big challenge. (Health Worker, Uganda)

In this and other similar situations the potential for effective knowledge mobilisation and systems impact was limited. This did not imply that knowledge was being exchanged but the resource and cultural environment restricted its benefit:

*Response*:   *"They shared knowledge especially when we asked them how they do it in their country. Comparing approaches and how they handle things".*

*Interviewer*: *"Do you think that knowledge could be applied here?"*

*Response*:   *"Not really, maybe. What is practical we can't do here. Here the patient comes and what we normally do is say what we think is right for them; which is wrong. Here patients don't even know their rights, they don't know what they are supposed to expect. There (in the UK) they say the patient has to be told all their options and they make a choice and if they don't want it that is ok; maybe that is a difference I saw. Here it may not be very practical for us because our patients don't even know what they are suffering from when they come. They don't know where to get information from so if we leave them to decide they may not do it; that is a limitation. The doctor will decide which medicine to give them and they take it; we convince them to take it but they really don't know what they are taking and sometimes they don't know the side effects but the patient should surely know before taking a drug they should expect the side effects."*

(Nurse, Uganda)

As this was a new placement group and we did not have long-term volunteers in this field we monitored this carefully and subsequently placed mental-health students with a mental-health specialist who runs a local NGO. We have noted above our reasons for not placing students outside of the public-health system. In some situations, where services are barely in existence or professions not yet developed this was the only option and the NGOs involved were actively interfacing with local public health facilities. This is certainly the case with the Youth and Women Foundation (YAWE).

## Case Study 4: The Youth and Women Foundation (YAWE) Mobile Clinic

For the reasons described above, K4C has partnered with the Youth and Women Foundation (YAWE).[19] YAWE focus on youth and gender empowerment with a particular emphasis on 'living positively' (with HIV). The Director of YAWE is a mental-health specialist. YAWE had been donated a mobile clinic to undertake community outreach work in rural villages and refugee camps. When we visited YAWE to discuss potential placements for mental-health nurses we found that the vehicle was not being used due to a lack of resource (fuel and manpower). We felt that the mobile clinic would offer unique opportunities for students and also critical complementary services in hard-to-reach areas. On that basis, we agreed to fund the costs of using the vehicle once or twice a month. During the outreach visits, local staff and the EEP students work alongside village health teams who mobilise the local community providing cervical screening, family planning, HIV diagnosis, care and treatment and diabetes screening alongside other public health services. The Director describes the value of these visits to his project and the local community:

> They do home visits – nursing care, malaria – wounds – those who need medication and also our mobile clinic they join the team when we go to the field – we provide fully fledged healthcare services including screening for HIV, diabetes because most people in the villages don't get the chance to get diagnoses because the equipment isn't there. The students from your program are very good – they do that – we provide them with strips – they

[19] www.yawefoundation.webs.com

also check BPs and cervical cancer screening but most of them have learnt that here because they come when they are not so skilled but they participate. They participate in the actual procedures.

When the team go out one of the professional volunteers usually accompanies them. The outreach clinics have proved particular attractive to placement students. As project managers, we were concerned that placing mental-health students at YAWE may put a burden on local staff. Whilst the supervisor admitted that hosting the students does imply an investment on his part he said he enjoys this and recognises the wider reciprocity involved:

> Interviewer: *"I was just trying to work out if you are making special plans distracting you from your normal work – are we making extra work for you?"*
>
> Response: *"It is true sometimes I feel they need attention especially the mental health students so I feel they benefit from having a person like me (a mental health specialist) with them so this week I have set up a program for them".*
>
> Interviewer: *"So you are doing extra work for the students?"*
>
> Response: *"Yes but they had a week of supervision and I wanted the students to see how mental health counsellors here work and what tools they use – how they diagnose here. Your project supports our outreaches (mobile clinic) so we are happy to help. I enjoy working with students and so long as it is planned it is OK".*

The final case study presented below is included as an example of project development and how students (in this case NHS Management Trainees) can be involved in quite strategic planning roles focused on some of the most serious obstacles to health systems change. This also illustrates the potential for multi-disciplinary integrated interventions engaging the kinds of knowledge clusters we referred to earlier on.

## CASE STUDY 5: BUILDING THE CASE FOR PUBLIC-PRIVATE-PARTNERSHIPS IN KABAROLE DISTRICT

As noted in Chapter 2, the EEP project was designed to provide placements for students. Most of the EEP participants have been studying at undergraduate level although many of them will already hold first degrees. Some of the students were also studying at Masters Level and several were involved in data collection for their doctorates.[20] Towards the end of the Health Education England project we were presented with an opportunity to organise a placement for NHS Management Trainees. These trainees are all graduates undertaking a fast-track management training with a view to becoming managers in the UK NHS. As a project, we were at the point of making a critical decision of whether to embark on a new project to restore functionality to a Health Centre IV facility that was failing to deliver effective maternity services.

Given our knowledge of this process and the very serious concerns we had about trying to get emergency obstetric services going in the absence of a doctor and our experience of trying to mobilise Ugandan doctors in these environments (Ackers et al. 2016) we mooted the idea of a Public-Private-Partnership drawing on a model explicitly advocated in the Ministry of Health Strategic Plan (2012). The success of this intervention, in our experience, rested on the ability to devolve the budget and responsibility for human and physical resource management to a PPP Management team. This represented an ambitious and entirely untested idea. The four NHS Management Trainees from the Central Manchester Foundation Trust were tasked to work alongside one of the project managers spending a month in Uganda to conduct a thorough scoping analysis and audit and prepare a proposal for a PPP intervention. The Trainees conducted some very high-quality work engaging in active negotiation and audit-related activity combined with interactions with local health workers to create the first steps in this potentially exciting new venture.[21]

## RELATIONSHIP AND CAPACITY-BUILDING IN PARTNER UNIVERSITIES

The EEP model involves another element of capacity-building that has been of great value to the local University and health system. The professional volunteers funded through the EEPs each co-teach one module on a new BSc Midwifery programme at Mountains of the Moon University (MMU). The programme was planned with considerable support from K4C and

---

[20] These students received funding from Santander.

[21] The outcome of this venture will not be clear for some time.

three professional volunteers and welcomed its first cohort of students in August 2015. It would have proved very difficult to get this programme off the ground in Uganda in the absence of professional volunteers as there are so few people qualified to teach the programme at degree level.[22] This model is focused on sustainability and capacity-building and co-presence in the teaching environment has been insisted upon in order to ensure that institutional memory and resources are built up for the future. The programme has also involved the active encouragement of MMU and diploma level midwives in selected local facilities to come to the UK to undertake recognised training programmes at Masters Level in order to build capacity in Uganda but also support mutual understanding of educational programmes and training systems. We have planned the whole process to focus on a small number of health centres which we are developing as established training sites both for UK and Ugandan students on placement (including Kagote). Whilst ensuring optimal learning outcomes for UK students this process has ensured that Ugandan students can begin to be supervised in fully functioning health facilities.

In some cases, the Ugandan fellows have been trained in research methods (rather than clinical areas) in order to build research capacity at MMU but also invest in the evaluation potential of our Ugandan colleagues. This will enable us in future to engage in genuine co-research activity. Asked to reflect on the contribution of the student placements to this area of activity the academic lead of Health Sciences responded;

[Is there anything we can do to improve to improve impact?]
   I've been very impressed with the quality of the students' teaching – of course they were mature students – but they did a really beautiful job teaching our students and our students really appreciate someone coming in and teaching them from outside (even if they are also students) they are teaching something appropriate to our student's environment and something practical too. I think it would be good to keep that in mind and plan ahead and make sure topics are needed to be covered – if

---

[22] Uganda faced a 'catch22' situation as the rules required that a degree programme in midwifery is taught by staff with a degree in midwifery. At the present time the number of midwives in Uganda with a degree can be counted on one hand.

we can think about it and plan ahead and the students are interested in teaching and it is good for them.

## CONCLUSIONS

The results of the EEP evaluation suggest that undergraduate placements can form the basis of valuable capacity-building work in low resource settings. We have been somewhat surprised at these results building as they do on several years' evaluation of the impact of far more experienced volunteers and the demand from host settings for the most senior and experienced professionals. Reflecting upon this apparent contradiction and the sense that student placements when organised in structured and deeply grounded 'knowledge clusters' may facilitate a higher level of sustainable systems change than the isolated deployment of highly qualified volunteers the logic is clear. The human resource environment in Uganda is such that for most of the time there are no doctors in situ and facilities are run by nurses, midwives and clinical/anaesthetic officers. The majority of staff in many facilities will be students themselves often at an early stage in their training with little concrete knowledge or experience and typically no effective supervision.

Referral systems are structurally damaged in the overwhelming majority of lower-level health facilities and basic neglected processes (patient monitoring; record keeping; audit; infection prevention control; and prescribing behaviour) are rarely in place. In these circumstances, we may question the merits of deploying highly qualified physicians to Uganda as they will rarely work in sustained co-present relationships with their peers. Deploying cadres of staff such as midwives and nurses facilities a more immediate engagement and the formation of highly effective training clusters supporting bi-lateral mentoring and knowledge exchange. This, coupled with the ability to identify and remove minor 'snagging' problems and leverage some conditionality within the local health system wherever possible through the fair-trade premium arguably constitutes the most efficient and effective intervention whilst also reducing the system destabilising effects associated with labour substitution UK students are far less likely to create the kinds of 'malignancy' referred to by Moyo (2009). The overall impact of EEPs is dampened by systems features and, most notably, staff absence and poor time-keeping. If staff are not presents and systems effectively close down in the afternoons then opportunities for knowledge mobilisation close down too. Responsibility here rests with the Uganda authorities to manage their human resource more effectively to improve motivation and reduce the need for moonlighting. An easy solution for placement providers would be to place students in better managed and remunerated private and mission facilities. As a project we do not believe that this 'solution' complies with ethical principles or gives the UK students the best understanding of global health.

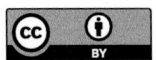

# CHAPTER 5

# Managing Reciprocity: No Harm Approaches to International Educational Placements

The idea of 'win-win' outcomes from international mobility is not new. Critiques of the 'brain drain' concept presented new hopes of mutually beneficial knowledge mobilisation referring to the returns to 'sending' countries via circulatory processes and virtual mobilities (Meyer 2003; Regets 2003). Our own work on scientific mobility concluded that brain drain as a concept was far too narrow and failed to capture the relationship between human mobility and knowledge mobilisation processes and the fact that mobility is the lifeblood of science in many resource starved regions (Ackers and Gill 2007). But these relationships are highly complex and there is no effective way of (quantitatively) 'measuring' losses and gains. To speak of win-win is to fail to capture these complexities and the critical importance of context to any evaluation of impact (Bate 2014). Our action-research study of ethical educational placements concludes that such exposures create transformational learning opportunities for the UK students involved. And these opportunities have the potential to make a significant contribution to the learning outcomes of direct relevance to curricula in their home universities. From the perspective of student learning we have no doubts that spending a period in a low resource setting is uniquely valuable. The learning premium and its specific relationship with core learning outcomes associated with academic study programmes will vary quite significantly depending on the structure and organisation of placements.

Placements organised through private sector companies capitalising on the swelling demand for volunteer-tourism, fuelled by university

© The Author(s) 2017
A. Ahmed et al., *The Ethics of Educational Healthcare Placements in Low and Middle Income Countries*, DOI 10.1007/978-3-319-48363-4_5

internationalisation processes, will generate some forms of useful learning. Taking students outside of their own country and the health systems they are accustomed to will necessarily develop systems thinking. It will push students out of their comfort zones and create opportunities for exposure to and reflection on cultural difference and global inequalities with the potential to build competence in global citizenship. Having said, that we have serious concerns that, unless placements are framed appropriately and adequate systems are in place to manage this process of intense engagement in a foreign environment there is a high risk that the 'shock' effects of what some authors have termed 'poverty tourism' (Dowell and Merrylees 2009)[1] could reinforce stereotypes. Simply being immersed in a low resource setting for four weeks and observing poverty does not necessarily translate into cultural competence. It may have quite the opposite effect. An important concern for placement providers here is to ensure a level of cultural awareness and understanding that goes beyond the potentially damaging effects of what Simpson calls the 'essentialized concepts of 'other' (2004: 682).

To the extent that international educational placements are just that: namely 'electives' (implying optional choices out with the core curriculum)[2] participation in forms of gap-year voluntourism provided by private companies may deliver valuable learning opportunities. And universities will (hopefully) pick up and challenge incidences of cultural 'mislearning' in reflective components of emerging global health curricula. We have serious doubts that such encounters generate the kind of curriculum-relevant learning that we have evidenced in the EEP project. Achieving this requires a much higher level of engagement that goes beyond quite voyeuristic 'observation-only' placements captured by Wearing and McGehee as a form of 'shallow volunteering' (2013: 123) and guards against the arrogance and risks associated with 'free mover'

---

[1] A shocking example of this has been described as 'orphanage tourism.' We have direct experience of the ways in which orphanages have been developed in Uganda as commodified 'honey pots' to attract gap-year students and the income associated with this 'market' creating new partnerships in corruption and opportunities for child abuse. For details, see http://www.thinkchildsafe.org/thinkbeforevisiting/

[2] Wikipedia defines 'An elective course is one chosen by a student from a number of optional subjects or courses in a curriculum, as opposed to a required course which the student must take' https://en.wikipedia.org/wiki/Course_(education)

medical electives. Achieving optimal curriculum and practice-relevant learning requires direct engagement with university programmes and effective supervision. When these structures are in place and embedded in active partnership working, international placements in low resource settings have the potential to become part of the core curriculum. This process of moving from 'out-of-program' electives to 'within–program' educational placements is important for a number of reasons. Firstly, because the learning returns in carefully planned and funded placements justify full recognition within education programmes. Secondly, because electives are inherently and increasingly associated with profound inequalities of opportunity. Notre Dame University defines electives as 'optional' but that does not imply free choice; the ability to access them has in the main reflected students' financial status (or that of their parents). As Wearing and McGehee note, most participants in international elective schemes have come from middle-class backgrounds (2013: 121).

Raymond and Hall go further suggesting that volunteer tourism exists in a highly commodified environment and serves as a 'stronghold for the privileged' (Raymond and Hall 2008). Social class and attitudes towards mobility are not a simple reflection of financial resource; they also reflect cultural or mobility 'capital'. Students who have been exposed to foreign travel at a younger age or for whom it has been a cultural expectation or rite of passage (as the medical elective often is) are far more likely to seek out elective placements and to process and manage the perceived risks involved. Most of the students who have taken part in the funded components of the EEPs are not in that situation and the EEP represents the first opportunity they have ever had to travel to a low resource setting. Certainly, most would not have taken this step without the encouragement and support of the project.

The funding provided by Health Education England coupled with the institutional support offered through the University of Salford-Knowledge for Change partnership facilitated these mobilities. The growing 'expectation of mobility' and the tendency for this to influence student opportunities and life chances at ever earlier stages in their education places pressure on education providers to recognise and respond to the inherent inequalities this presents. One of the major providers of placements, 'Work the World' advertises its dentistry placements with the strapline: 'A specialist dentistry placement with us will set you apart from anyone who chose to play it safe and stay in the UK'.[3] The website advertises placements at a basic cost of £1390 for four weeks (plus £300 registration fee) excluding international flights making a placement cost in the region of £2300. Another provider (Projects Abroad)[4] provide a price list depending on the location and type of placements to around £1,800 (for four weeks) taking the price including flights, and visas to over £2500. These are far cheaper than many other providers with students reporting costs of over £4000 for elective placements often with an additional expectation of donations attached. As Hartman et al. describe, higher education and volunteering represent the largest growth sectors in the youth and tourism industry in a market which they estimate to be worth over 2 billion dollars globally. Wearing and McGehee in their review of the burgeoning literature on 'volunteer tourism' cite figures suggesting that volunteer tourists spend between £838m and £1.3b per year (2013: 120).

An international placement is not an 'elective' if a student cannot afford to access it or lacks the confidence to engage. Bringing placements in-programme renders the inequalities explicit and forces key actors in universities and the NHS to recognise and respond to them. The process will also put pressure on private providers engaged in the commodification of placements to show value-for-money. It will also expose the genuine costs of this form of activity to universities enabling them to consider their role in the new fees structure for nursing, midwifery and allied health professions and the possibility of developing equitable ways of managing these to an increasingly diverse student body.

So far, we have discussed the benefits of international placements to the students in 'sending' countries and the potential costs involved raising issues of equity and quality. When ethics are raised in the context of placements the discussion is usually with the impacts on 'host' settings. Most of the private providers offering placements pay at least lip service to the development impacts of placements typically referring to either cash payments or donations as forms of compensatory 'payments' in this commodified environment. By way of example 'Work the World'[5] advertise

---

[3] http://www.worktheworld.co.uk/dentistry-electives
[4] http://projects-abroad.co.uk/
[5] See note 3.

the 'support for partners' offered through their schemes stating that, 'we make a point of recognising [our supervising staff] by financially rewarding them, personally, for their efforts'. Furthermore, 'a fixed sum is given to each and every hospital for every student we send'. They go on to show photographs of huge volumes of consumables donated to facilities and to list equipment donations. Whilst it is important not to underplay the potential value of these forms of compensation each component of this raises serious concerns to anyone with a knowledge and understanding of working in low resource settings.

## Reciprocity and Fair Trade Learning

In 2016, FK Norway[6] commissioned an international expert Benjamin Lough to draft a report setting out the Norwegian model of 'international volunteer service' recasting volunteers as agents of change working in more equitable and balanced relationships with their partners in host countries. The report identifies reciprocity as the core value guiding the ethics of these exchanges. In line with the critiques of more traditional donor-recipient models of 'volunteering' it acknowledges the fundamental asymmetry responsible for the dependencies and harms associated with professional voluntarism. Citing Polonijo-King (2004) Lough refers to concerns that 'unidirectional aid relationships ultimately rob recipients of self-respect using altruism as a form of social oppression' (p.109). He goes on to propose that 'reciprocal learning is one expression of strategic reciprocity [ … ] disrupting the helping narrative' (p10). This resonates with our own experience of managing EEPs. The concept of 'student' is far more balanced than that of 'volunteer' and enables local hosts to conceptualise themselves as active participants in an exchange relationship rather than as the passive recipients of foreign 'expertise'. These forms of symbiosis are most evident in engagements involving not only academic partners (as traditional student exchanges) but also service or non-academic partners. Sharpe and Dear (2013) use the concept of 'International Service-Learning' or 'ISL' to describe

---

[6] FK Norway is a part of the Norwegian national developmental policy. It was established in 1963 to send people from Norway, and was reorganised in 2000 to do mutual exchange: http://www.fredskorpset.no/en/about-us/

university programmes in the US that 'combine academic instruction and community service in an international context' (2013: 49). The ISL approach has more in common with our concept of Ethical Educational Placements than the commodified products offered to consumers of volunteer tourism. In addition to the kinds of 'person-to-person' reciprocity evident in the relationships that mobile students have with their peers and health workers, Lough underlines the role of organisational reciprocity in supporting effective and balanced interventions.

A critical component of the success of the EEP model lies in the partnerships that underpin and operationalise it. According to Wearing and McGehee the organisations that engage in the operation of volunteer tourism are a key factor in maximising good practice (2013: 124). Knowledge for Change (K4C) as a social enterprise plays a critical brokerage function linking key stakeholders including the University of Salford, Mountains of the Moon University, Uganda and Kabarole Health District. Hartman et al. argue that the 'unique mission, research, and evaluation capacities of higher education' places universities centre stage in the university-community nexus facilitating opportunities for 'best practice' maximising the benefits and minimising the negative impacts for host communities and volunteers. Whilst we would prefer to see the EEP model as conveying ethical standards for educational placements (as opposed to volunteer tourism) we would concur with their view that universities have institutional characteristics which make them 'ideal catalysts' (p. 109) for change. These typically include a not-for profit foundation; public serving missions with a focus on education, academic expertise in research, a research-based understanding of international development and an inherent commitment to challenging inequality, dependency and injustice. Wearing and McGehee refer in their review of the literature on volunteer tourism, a shift towards a more 'scientific' critique of the phenomenon involving more structured, interdisciplinary, transnational and mixed-methods studies (2013: 122).[7] All of the organisations involved must also commit to principals of *good governance* and the

---

[7] They couch this discussion as lying at the intersection of tourism and volunteering research; we would argue that there are other perhaps more insightful theoretical insights to be had here from studies of mobility and internationalisation in higher education and careers.

promotion of transparency and accountability.[8] This is the cornerstone of trust and trust lies at the heart of partnership relationships.

The University partners in the EEP pilot provide important support and credibility to educational placements. Salford University, by way of example, underwrites the risk assessment process drawing on significant expertise in placement management. As a not-for-profit organisation committed to education and training it provides a level of credibility for potential students seeking out placement opportunities that is not found amongst private sector companies. The EEP secretariat is firmly based in Salford's prestigious Knowledge and Place Research Group ensuring a firm grounding in research on internationalisation processes, global health and research/evaluation methodology. As such EEPs represent a prime example of evidence-based policy. The University also supports high level dissemination of the EEP model encouraging other placement providers to reflect on their programmes and consider whether they can improve on the learning environment and ensure that they comply with ethical principles. The Universities in Uganda provide a similar assurance of support for students when on placement and a focus on learning and knowledge exchange. Working with these partners opens unique opportunities for peer-peer co-working but also harnesses and facilitates the role that Community Universities (such as MMU) play in delivering training to health workers in their hinterland. The link with Kabarole District is also essential to ensure that proper systems are in place and senior managers are aware of the presence and activities of volunteers and students. Also that they are given the opportunity to discuss and negotiate those interventions creating new opportunities and minimising the potential for unintended consequences. Once these relationships are established and respected K4C can then operate at a more detailed level in the negotiation of specific tailored placements linked into active on-going project interventions with key actors within the District including health facilities and collaborating partners. An effective and respected intermediary with the capacity to manage relationships and maintain a close understanding of context is critical to this process. The intermediary also plays an essential role in managing and mitigating risk and operationalising the risk assessment process which is necessarily fluid and reactive.

---

[8] Governance is identified as one of the cornerstone principles of Fair Trade: http://www.fairtrade.org.uk/en/what-is-fairtrade/the-impact-of-our-work/our-theory-of-change

On another level the intermediary organisation has a fundamental role to play in ensuring compliance with ethical principles. As with risk, ethical compliance is an on-going process involving constant negotiation and mediation. The issues are complex and confounded by the innovative dynamics of global inequalities and corruption. Every intervention generates externality effects (unintended consequences) many of which are difficult to predict.

## THE MULTIPLIER EFFECTS OF STUDENT CONSUMPTION

Chapter 4 identified a number of ways in which EEPs have made a sustainable impact on local health systems in Uganda through the 'Fair Trade Premium'. We did not include in that discussion the wider economic impacts associated with students as consumers in local economies. However, anyone who has been involved in touristic activities in Uganda will see how important students and volunteers are to local tourism; the majority of participants in touristic visits in Uganda are volunteers or students often undertaking tourism alongside other activities. Hartman et al. extend their concept of Fair Trade Learning to consumption behaviour suggesting that programmes should take care to use 'local eateries' and source local products including local guides. We would support that assertion and have taken strides to discourage donations of equipment from the UK preferring wherever possible to source medical equipment in-country. We have been fortunate to have the intelligence and connections of our sister bio-medical engineering project to support us in this work. An example of this can be seen in the endeavours of a group of returned students actively wishing to continue their involvement in Uganda and respond to an identified need (for cervical cancer treatment). The students had taken part in the YAWE cervical screening work (Case Study 4) but were concerned that many women who were tested positive then had to make a 5–6 hour journey to Kampala for (potential) treatment. They therefore decided on return to raise funds for a cryotherapy machine to co-develop a local service. K4C became involved in this taking advice from the biomedical engineering project and seeking in the first instance to procure equipment from Uganda providers. Having researched the situation, we have decided to source an alternative machine not yet available in Uganda but less reliant upon expensive consumables. K4C have since agreed to support this service providing the engineering and clinical training with the support of our long-term volunteers to ensure the equipment functions effectively for a minimum of three years.

Hartman et al. also advocate the use of host families in the host setting to accommodate students. This is something we have chosen as a project not to engage in for a number of reasons. The students on EEPs are first and foremost professionals and not tourists and, on that basis, we feel it is important that they do not live with local families. From a risk perspective, we have preferred to organise our own premises and ensure that students have access to the facilities they need to maintain contact with their home universities and families. Many of the EEP students are mature students with partners and children and many continue to engage in elements of coursework during their placements. We also ask them to prepare teaching materials and weekly reports and prefer to provide them with the facilities to do that. Students on placement in the UK would not live with local families and we do not feel this contributes to their professional identity and external perceptions of them as students on educational placements. We have also found that students faced with quite challenging placements need to connect together in the evenings to debrief and share experiences with their peers, placement managers and supervisors. Having said that we have engaged our sister project (OBAAT)[9] to undertake all of the building and repairs work using local builders engaged in capacity-building construction projects.

Sharpe and Dear's evaluation of 'International Service-Learning' (2013) echoes our own experiences and the importance of understanding the messiness of these kinds of interventions and the constant contradictions and unintended consequences muddying relationships between project rhetoric and practical reality. We present the EEP model in this book not as a static and perfectly formed 'model' but as a work in progress representing at least a commitment to progressive practice if not its complete realisation. The journey continues as we constantly try new things and reflect upon them. What is of utmost importance is that we continue to build upon our evidence base to improve the quality of the concept and its execution and, as Hartman et al. advocate, 'move forward in a sector increasingly dominated by a noxious combination of slick marketing and under-informed consumers'.

The emphasis on community-engagement and multi-disciplinarity in Hartman's 'Fair Trade Learning' has been taken a step further in our current plans to develop a series of integrated multi-disciplinary group

[9] See note 53.

projects in line with Salford University's employability agenda.[10] The plans for these placements follows similar lines to the existing EEP model but with greater emphasis on the identification of a specific need or project by local stakeholders and the recruitment of explicitly multi-disciplinary student teams to support an intervention. By way of illustration, one of the projects we are currently recruiting to involves a planned relationship between the Ugandan and UK Blood Transfusion Services designed to reduce mortality and morbidities associated with poor access to blood. The supply of blood in Uganda is constrained by a whole range of factors including donor awareness and behaviour, the lack of capacity in equipment management and repair, lack of capacity in laboratory management and skills and problems with power (to supply cold chain networks) and transportation. There is also no capacity in Uganda at the present time for cell salvage to enable patients to receive their own blood during operations taking the pressure off donor blood supplies, reducing costs and improving safety. The problems call for multi-disciplinary complex interventions involving many different stakeholders and all kinds of knowledge. We hope that the kinds of knowledge clusters generated within the EEP programme will enable us to mount an effective if incremental approach to such challenges.

## EARLY CAREER MOBILITY AND GLOBAL CITIZENSHIP

All studies of student mobility concur on one thing; that early stage mobility is an important precursor of subsequent mobility. We have expressed some concerns (above) that the kinds of mobility associated with 'electives' has been largely restricted, until recent years, to the mobilities of the privileged and noted that this reflects not solely income differentials but also differences in life experiences and exposure to mobility in their lives. One of the key findings of the EEP study has been the confidence and thirst the opportunity has given to young people with little previous experience or perhaps even interest in global health to consider future visits. It is interesting to see how cadres of students who would have had little opportunity to spend time in a low resource setting subsequently talk about their futures. We have referred to the specific challenges of

[10] We have received funding to develop and pilot these through Salford University's Higher Education Innovation Fund (HEIF).

placing students in cadres that do not even exist in Uganda. This hasn't stopped one of the podiatry students planning to work abroad in future. Interestingly she also talks very positively about the attractiveness of multidisciplinary working:

> I'm so glad I did it, and it's helped me realise what I want to do future and I know that I want to work abroad. It's made it a lot clearer. It's helped me realise what type of thing I want to go into. I want to work with high-risk things and with multidisciplinary areas.

Another student, this time in prosthetics also expresses a desire to plan a longer stay in a low resource setting in future:

> Even though we weren't there for too long, we felt like we made a big difference in people's lives. It has definitely given me the motivation to do something like this again. I have always wanted to do some care relief work in developing countries, and I definitely will now, even if it's just for a couple of years.

The final section summarises the key ingredients of the Ethical Educational Placement Model.

## EEP MODEL

### *Infrastructure Investment Through Partnership-Building*

*Sending Organisations*
Phase 1 requires the establishment of 'Fit-For-Purpose' Sending Organisations.

Ideally these would involve a combination of a Registered Charity (NGO)[11] working in partnership with a Higher Education Institution (with not-for-profit and explicit educational objectives).

Identification of key managerial roles in sending and receiving locations (to include an overall Project Manager and Placement Leads in both locations). Individuals in these roles need a firm grounding in the

---

[11] We note in Ackers and Ackers Johnson (2016) the importance of these organisations operating within the spirit and letter of UK equality law.

context and capacity-building objectives. It is essential not to underestimate the level of commitment and investment required to ensure that individuals with the right level of knowledge and skills are employed in these positions. **Financial Planning and Transparency** is essential.

### Host Organisations

This includes the identification and formation of firm trust and governance relationships with partners[12] in the hosting setting established through continuous collaboration. Ideally these would involve local HEIs partnership with relevant local stakeholders. From an ethical perspective we would advocate working only within the frame of public services and those NGOs committed to supporting pubic services.

Where appropriate objective setting processes and objectives should be formalised through a Memorandum of Understanding or similar agreement. This needs to be a 'living' document responsive to the outcomes of evaluation (below) with periodic review built in.

### Professional Volunteers

Deployment of Professional Volunteers to support Partnership capacity-building objectives. The EEP Volunteer Agreement combines capacity-building roles in PUBLIC facilities with co-teaching in HEIs and placement supervision (of UK and Local students in knowledge clusters).[13]

### Placement Operationalisation

Once infrastructure and active partnership working with established goals are in place planning can commence for placements.

Where possible ethical educational placements should be **Integrated within Undergraduate Curricula** rather than sitting outside of them in the form of 'electives'. This should expose them to full interrogation from

---

[12] This could be a Health Partnership or a partnership with local schools, for example.

[13] Further details of Professional Volunteer deployment and Volunteer Agreements are provided in Ackers et al. (2016) and Ackers and Ackers-Johnson (2016).

equality and ethical perspectives and ensure that curriculum-relevant learning is actively validated.

This requires attention to undergraduate curricula to ensure a firm grounding in **Ethics and Global Health /International Development in Undergraduate Curricula** (including cultural competence) for ALL students.[14]

**Comprehensive and Fair Recruitment** processes complying with best practice in equal opportunities including maximum exposure to opportunities available, open advertisement of opportunities and rigorous selection criteria (where bursaries are involved). Clear procedures re disclosure of health and other conditions to ensure that all students have the necessary resilience to cope with a placement and team-working.

Comprehensive and tailored approach to **Pre-departure Training and Induction**; ideally combining provision of regularly up-dated Induction and Orientation materials with opportunities for one-on-one email and face-to-face communication. To include expectations management. Where possible, engagement of host partners in this process.

The Induction Pack should contain links to full **Risk Assessment** and a bespoke and comprehensive **Insurance Policy.** Wherever possible students (and Professional Volunteers) should be covered by a Common Policy to ensure rapid and effective response to crises and ensure there are no gaps in cover.

Centrally planned and clearly communicated logistical arrangements need to be in place to ensure the management of student journeys from initial expression of interest to final post-return reporting/reflection. Particular attention to in-country travel, provision of risk-assessed accommodation with amenities necessary for completion of an effective and professional *educational* placement (this will vary according the local context). Provision of services of a **Local Placement Manager** actively engaged within the overall Partnership activity (as above). The local placement manager will work alongside Professional Volunteers and project managers to ensure effective debriefing and pastoral care.

---

[14] This is an area that we are currently working on and was not fully established prior to deployment of EEP students. The research has suggested this is necessary to prepare students and promote optimal learning and guard against the concerns expressed about 'essentialized concepts of 'other' (Simpson cited in Chapter 5).

Establishment of a **Placement Agreement** providing generic clarity on student roles on placement, codes of conduct (including disciplinary procedures), co-presence and supervision/mentoring with an additional tailored component specific to each individual student. This should be seen as an iterative agreement established prior to departure but subject to negotiated revision during the placement in response to changing needs and contexts.

Financial planning and governance requirements (above) extend to the relationships with local hosts and the management of the **Fair Trade Premium**. Serious consideration should be given to any cash payments and avoided wherever possible. Local stakeholders should be actively involved at the appropriate level where possible involving local health workers in decisions about local investments to support joint decision-making and effective outcomes.

### *Evaluation and Iterative Review*

Integrated Evaluation of the wider capacity-building initiative and within that, the Placement Review. This is as an on-going requirement to ensure that all of the above are adhered to and optimal outcomes achieved (including attention to 'no harm' principles). Placement review and reporting should include written weekly reports and focus group meetings supported, where necessary, by opportunities for personal discussions with the Local Placement Manager.

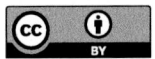

# APPENDIX 1

## ETHICAL EDUCATIONAL PLACEMENT STUDENT AGREEMENT

This agreement contains placement details, a code of conduct and outlines project evaluation requirements. Please read through fully and carefully before signing and returning to the project manager. No student/volunteer will be allowed to begin their placement until the agreement has been signed and returned.

### USUAL PLACEMENT HOURS AND LEAVE

- Students are expected to 'work' for an average of 37 hours per week whilst on placement.
- Students are expected to 'work' regular hours each day. The timing of these hours can be discussed with the project manager and may be subject to flexibility. They may include night placements or weekends if necessary, provided that the co-presence principle is always respected.
- Students may spend their evenings and weekends as they please (within certain limitations).
- Students will be required to advise the Project Manager of where they are travelling to if moving outside of Fort Portal during the placement. No student will be allowed to travel outside of Uganda during their placements without prior written consent from the Project Manager.

© The Author(s) 2017                                                                131
A. Ahmed et al., *The Ethics of Educational Healthcare Placements in Low and Middle Income Countries*, DOI 10.1007/978-3-319-48363-4

## STUDENT CONDUCT

Students are reminded that whilst they are in Uganda they are representing Knowledge for Change, the University of Salford and their own University and/or professional body. Students are required to behave in a manner that reflects the professional standing of both the UK institutions and the host organisations in Uganda.

Students are required to adhere to the risk assessment guidance. Any deviation from the risk assessment guidance may imply a breach of the terms of their insurance. Students should be aware that if they do deviate from the assessment/guidance that they do so at their own risk.

Any behaviour that brings Knowledge for Change, the University of Salford, or any of our partner organisations into disrepute will be dealt with through the University of Salford Disciplinary Policy.

Policies and rules relating to student conduct are necessary to support the efficient and smooth running of the Educational Placement Project. It is acknowledged that the majority of students consistently behave appropriately. However, it is necessary that a disciplinary procedure is available which is understood by all and outlines the rights and obligations of students and managers to ensure that fairness and equity are applied in all circumstances.

This document applies to all students and/or volunteers participating in either short or long stay programmes. The guidelines within this document also apply to medical students and short-term volunteers participating in the link during their placement module and any medical staff volunteering in Uganda as part of the Educational Placement Project.

The following are examples of offences that, having given due consideration to all of the circumstances, may be regarded by the University of Salford as *Gross Misconduct*. It is possible that a student could be dis missed without previous warnings. This list is indicative. It is not to be regarded as exclusive or exhaustive:

- Misuse of drugs, for example through misappropriation of drugs or being under the influence of illicit drugs.
- Criminal conduct while participating in the Educational Placement Project.
- Sexual offences or sexual misconduct while participating in the Educational Placement Project.

- Conduct likely to offend decency (employees need to be aware and observe cultural differences).
- Violence or other exceptionally offensive behaviour.
- Discrimination against a member of staff or public on the grounds of sex, race, colour, nationality, marital status, sexual orientation, religion, disability or social background.
- Breaches of safety regulations endangering oneself or other people including deliberate damage to, neglect of, or misappropriation of safety equipment. Reckless behaviour which constitutes a danger to health or safety of any person.
- Breaches of confidentiality relating to patients, staff or other persons.

Listed below are examples of offences of **Misconduct**, other than gross misconduct, which may result in disciplinary action and/or counselling in the light of the circumstances of each case. This list is to be regarded neither as exclusive nor exhaustive. Other forms of misconduct may give rise to disciplinary action.

- When a member of the team fails to observe, without sufficient cause, operational regulations while participating in the Educational Placement Project.
- Where any member of the team renders himself/herself unfit, through the use of alcohol or illicit drugs, for duties which he/she is, or will be required to perform, or which he/she may reasonably foresee having to perform. For example, unfit to conduct project work due to use of drink/drugs on the previous day/night.
- Smoking within the work place or in public areas or while in the company of community officials, local workers and patients (this can cause offence in Africa). This also includes smoking within student accommodation and surrounding areas.
- Failure by any member of the team to adhere to the risk assessment guidelines without good reason.

## Project Evaluation and Review

Evaluation of individual progress is a process designed to form a rolling record of your experience and learning in Uganda. It is also an essential component of Project Evaluation. All students /volunteers must comply with the Project Evaluation processes designed by Knowledge for Change and the University of Salford which may include interviews, focus groups and written reports/blogs. You may also wish to develop a personal or public blog detailing the activity on your placements, but please be aware of ethical aspects and confidentiality.

## DECLARATION

In signing the Placement Agreement; you are acknowledging that you have read and understood the content within the Agreement, the Induction Pack, the Risk Assessment document and Travel/Medical Insurance documentation. You are also agreeing that you have undergone any necessary health checks, are up to date on all required inoculations, have made arrangements to ensure you have a supply of anti-malarials for the duration of your placement, and will comply with the University of Salford's project evaluation activities.

**Student name:**
**Student number:**
**University:**
**Date:**
**Signature:**

# Appendix 2

## The Ethical Elective Placement Project – Post-Placement Student Survey

The post-placement survey was created using SurveyMonkey software and was sent to all students who completed placements as part of the Ethical Elective Placement project. The survey was circulated by WhatsApp using a web link in October 2016. Of the 111 students it was sent to, it was only received by 104, suggesting that 7 of the students had either did not have access to WhatsApp or had changed their contact details in the time between completing their placements and being sent the survey. WhatsApp was used as a medium for dissemination of the survey link as many of the students had graduated by the time the survey was circulated and would be unlikely to still have access to their university emails accounts. It was also expected to provide a higher response rate due to the nature of the technology and the age range of the students.

Sixty-five students completed the survey in total, representing a response rate of 59% of all the students who completed a placement, or 63% of those students who received the link. It comprised seven primary questions, the results for which are listed below (Fig. A.1):

© The Author(s) 2017
A. Ahmed et al., *The Ethics of Educational Healthcare Placements in Low and Middle Income Countries*, DOI 10.1007/978-3-319-48363-4

## Which University course were/are you studying?

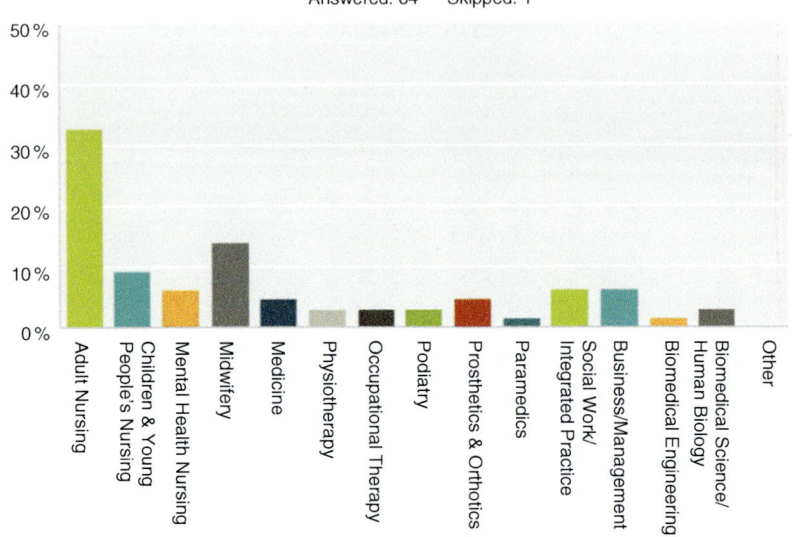

Answered: 64    Skipped: 1

| Answer Choices | Responses | |
|---|---|---|
| Adult Nursing | 32.81% | 21 |
| Children & Young People's Nursing | 9.38% | 6 |
| Mental Health Nursing | 6.25% | 4 |
| Midwifery | 14.06% | 9 |
| Medicine | 4.69% | 3 |
| Physiotherapy | 3.13% | 2 |
| Occupational Therapy | 3.13% | 2 |
| Podiatry | 3.13% | 2 |
| Prosthetics & Orthotics | 4.69% | 3 |
| Paramedics | 1.56% | 1 |
| Social Work/Integrated Practice | 6.25% | 4 |
| Business/Management | 6.25% | 4 |
| Biomedical Engineering | 1.56% | 1 |
| Biomedical Science/Human Biology | 3.13% | 2 |
| Other (Please Specify) | 0.00% | 0 |
| Total | | 64 |

**Fig. A.1**    Questions 1–5

## In which country did you complete your electric placement?

Answered: 65     Skipped: 0

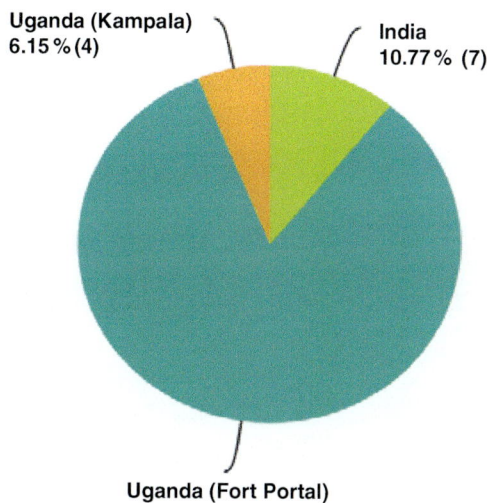

Uganda (Kampala)
6.15 % (4)

India
10.77 % (7)

Uganda (Fort Portal)

| Answer Choices | Responses | |
|---|---|---|
| India | 10.77% | 7 |
| Uganda (Fort Portal) | 83.08% | 54 |
| Uganda (Kampala) | 6.15% | 4 |
| **Total** | | **65** |

**Fig. A.1**   (continued)

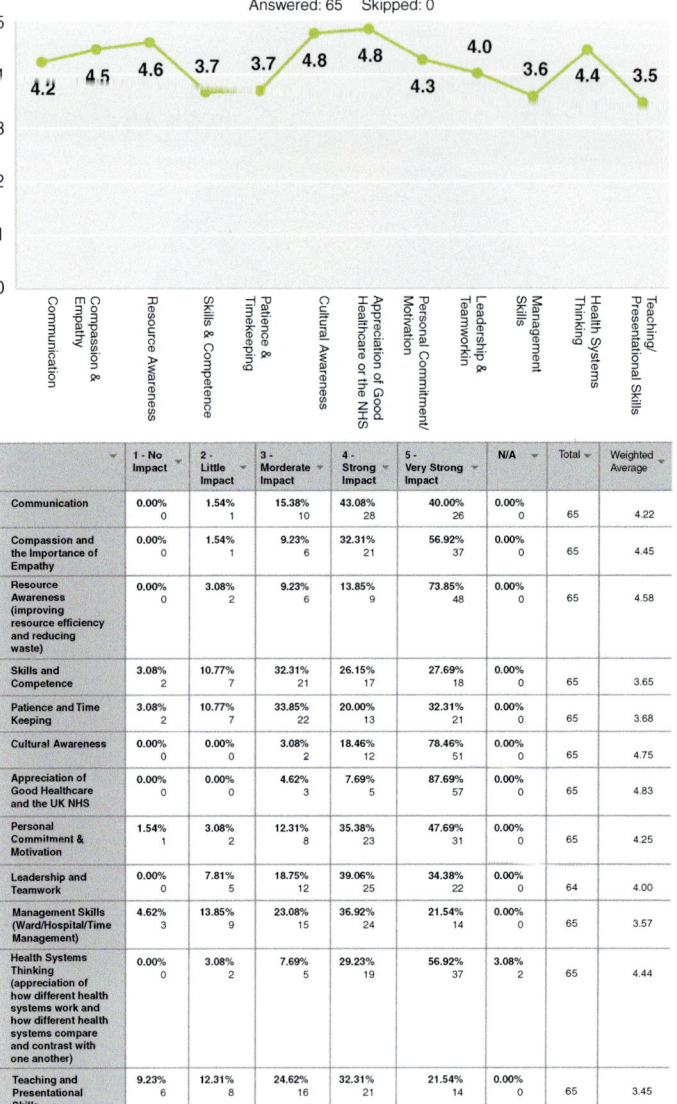

**What impact did the placement have on your learning in each of the following areas?**

Answered: 65    Skipped: 0

| | 1 - No Impact | 2 - Little Impact | 3 - Morderate Impact | 4 - Strong Impact | 5 - Very Strong Impact | N/A | Total | Weighted Average |
|---|---|---|---|---|---|---|---|---|
| Communication | 0.00% <br> 0 | 1.54% <br> 1 | 15.38% <br> 10 | 43.08% <br> 28 | 40.00% <br> 26 | 0.00% <br> 0 | 65 | 4.22 |
| Compassion and the Importance of Empathy | 0.00% <br> 0 | 1.54% <br> 1 | 9.23% <br> 6 | 32.31% <br> 21 | 56.92% <br> 37 | 0.00% <br> 0 | 65 | 4.45 |
| Resource Awareness (improving resource efficiency and reducing waste) | 0.00% <br> 0 | 3.08% <br> 2 | 9.23% <br> 6 | 13.85% <br> 9 | 73.85% <br> 48 | 0.00% <br> 0 | 65 | 4.58 |
| Skills and Competence | 3.08% <br> 2 | 10.77% <br> 7 | 32.31% <br> 21 | 26.15% <br> 17 | 27.69% <br> 18 | 0.00% <br> 0 | 65 | 3.65 |
| Patience and Time Keeping | 3.08% <br> 2 | 10.77% <br> 7 | 33.85% <br> 22 | 20.00% <br> 13 | 32.31% <br> 21 | 0.00% <br> 0 | 65 | 3.68 |
| Cultural Awareness | 0.00% <br> 0 | 0.00% <br> 0 | 3.08% <br> 2 | 18.46% <br> 12 | 78.46% <br> 51 | 0.00% <br> 0 | 65 | 4.75 |
| Appreciation of Good Healthcare and the UK NHS | 0.00% <br> 0 | 0.00% <br> 0 | 4.62% <br> 3 | 7.69% <br> 5 | 87.69% <br> 57 | 0.00% <br> 0 | 65 | 4.83 |
| Personal Commitment & Motivation | 1.54% <br> 1 | 3.08% <br> 2 | 12.31% <br> 8 | 35.38% <br> 23 | 47.69% <br> 31 | 0.00% <br> 0 | 65 | 4.25 |
| Leadership and Teamwork | 0.00% <br> 0 | 7.81% <br> 5 | 18.75% <br> 12 | 39.06% <br> 25 | 34.38% <br> 22 | 0.00% <br> 0 | 64 | 4.00 |
| Management Skills (Ward/Hospital/Time Management) | 4.62% <br> 3 | 13.85% <br> 9 | 23.08% <br> 15 | 36.92% <br> 24 | 21.54% <br> 14 | 0.00% <br> 0 | 65 | 3.57 |
| Health Systems Thinking (appreciation of how different health systems work and how different health systems compare and contrast with one another) | 0.00% <br> 0 | 3.08% <br> 2 | 7.69% <br> 5 | 29.23% <br> 19 | 56.92% <br> 37 | 3.08% <br> 2 | 65 | 4.44 |
| Teaching and Presentational Skills | 9.23% <br> 6 | 12.31% <br> 8 | 24.62% <br> 16 | 32.31% <br> 21 | 21.54% <br> 14 | 0.00% <br> 0 | 65 | 3.45 |

**Fig. A.1**  (continued)

## How relevent to your University Course was the experience and learning you achieved during your placement?

Answered: 65    Skipped: 0

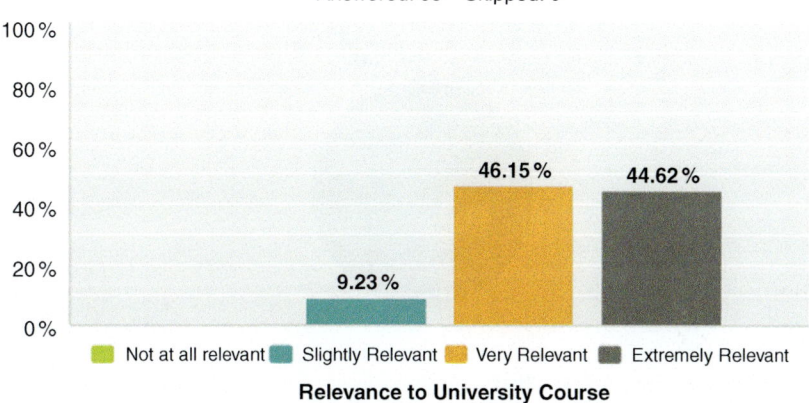

**Relevance to University Course**

| Answer Choices | Responses | |
|---|---|---|
| Not at all Relevant | 0.00% | 0 |
| Slightly Relevant | 9.23% | 6 |
| Very Relevant | 46.15% | 30 |
| Extremely Relevant | 44.62% | 29 |
| **Total** | | **65** |

**Fig. A.1**   (continued)

**What do you think impact of completing the placement will be on your future career and employability?**

Answered: 64    Skipped: 1

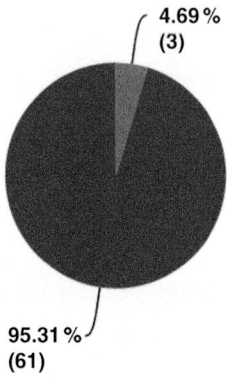

4.69%
(3)

95.31%
(61)

| Answer Choices | Responses | |
|---|---|---|
| Very Negative | 0.00% | 0 |
| Slightly Negative | 0.00% | 0 |
| No Impact | 0.00% | 0 |
| Slightly Positive | 4.69% | 3 |
| Very Positive | 95.31% | 61 |
| **Total** | | **64** |

**Fig. A.1** (continued)

## Overall, what impact do you believe your placement  had on the individuals/facilities/organisations/health system in the country within which you were placed?

Answered: 65   Skipped: 0

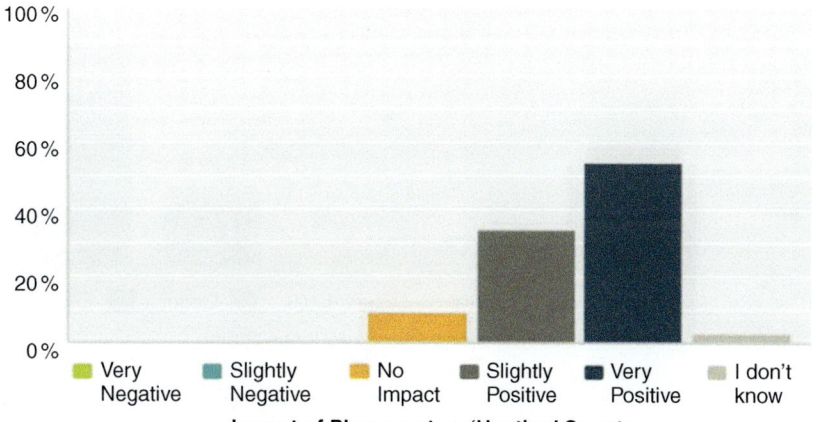

Impact of Placement on 'Hosting' Country

| Answer Choices | Responses | |
|---|---|---|
| Very Negative | 0.00% | 0 |
| Slightly Negative | 0.00% | 0 |
| No Impact | 9.23% | 6 |
| Slightly Positive | 33.85% | 22 |
| Very Positive | 53.85% | 35 |
| I Don't Know | 3.08% | 2 |
| **Total** | | **65** |

**Fig. A.1**   (continued)

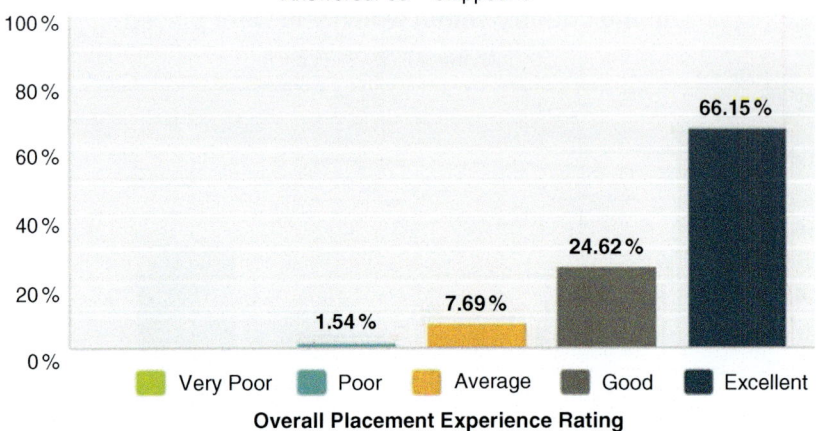

**How would you rate your overall placement experience?**

Answered: 65   Skipped: 0

**Overall Placement Experience Rating**

| Answer Choices | Responses | |
|---|---|---|
| Very Poor | 0.00% | 0 |
| Poor | 1.54% | 1 |
| Average | 7.69% | 5 |
| Good | 24.62% | 16 |
| Excellent | 66.15% | 43 |
| **Total** | | **65** |

**Fig. A.1**   (continued)

# Appendix 3

# Interview Schedule

International Placements, Uganda. Pre-departure
interview schedule: students

Preamble: Purpose of interview, confidentiality, anonymity (Fig. A.2).

1. Placement Experience

   a. Can you describe/tell me a little bit about what you did on your placement?
   b. What specifically did you gain from the placement in terms of your study and work? What skills and knowledge did you learn/apply in your study and work?
   c. What specifically did you gain/learn from the placement beyond study and work?
   d. What do you think you contributed to your placement hosts?
   e. What were the main challenges for you on the placement, if any? (personal, social, academic/professional)

2. The Placement: Structure and Support

   a. Looking back, do you feel you were prepared for your placement? What did you find most/least helpful?
   b. What kind of information or training (or support) do you think volunteers or students might benefit from that you haven't had?

© The Author(s) 2017                                                              143
A. Ahmed et al., *The Ethics of Educational Healthcare Placements in Low
and Middle Income Countries*, DOI 10.1007/978-3-319-48363-4

| Biographical/study background data (if not previously collected during pre-interview) | |
|---|---|
| Name (interviewee) | |
| Year of birth | |
| Sex | Male ☐ <br><br> Female ☐ |
| Ethnicity | |
| Nationality | |
| Relationship status | Single ☐ <br><br> Relationship (not co-habiting) ☐ <br><br> Live-in partner/spouse ☐ |
| Caring responsibilities | Children ☐    Other ☐ |
| Work outside study | No ☐    Yes part time ☐    Yes full time ☐ |
| Volunteering activities | Yes ☐    No ☐ |
| Course level | undergraduate ☐    postgraduate ☐ |
| Course name | |
| Course year | 1 ☐    2 ☐    3 ☐    4 ☐ <br><br> (Is this the final year?  Yes ☐ No ☐) |
| Funding for placement | Self ☐    HEE ☐    Bursary ☐ <br><br> Other ☐  Please specify _____ ) |

**Fig. A.2**  Questionnaire

    c. How easy/difficult was it for you to take part in the placement? How did you manage/cope in the context of other aspects of your life? (work, study, family etc.)?

    d. How do you feel about the supervision of your placement?

    e. What about accommodation /travel/food etc.?

    f. Length of stay?

3. Final Question

    a. In terms of your learning, can you tell me a bit about how it relates to your course and the learning outcomes associated with that?

    b. How do you feel this may add to your CV/future employability?

    c. Could you in a few words sum up how you are feeling about the placement now?

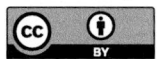

# References

Ackerman, L. K. (2010). The ethics of short-term international health electives in developing countries. *Annals of Behavioural Science and Medical Education,* *16*(2), 40–43.

Ackers, H. L. (2015). Mobilities and knowledge transfer: Understanding the contribution of volunteer stays to North-South healthcare partnerships'. *International Migration, 53*(1), 131–147.

Ackers, H. L., & Ackers-Johnson, J. (2016). *Mobile professional voluntarism and international development: Killing me softly?* New York: Palgrave.

Ackers, H. L., & Gill, B. (2007). *Moving people and knowledge: Scientific mobility in an enlarged European Union.* London: Edward Elgar.

Ackers, H. L., Ioannou, E., & Ackers-Johnson, J. (2016). The impact of delays on maternal and neonatal outcomes in Ugandan public health facilities: The role of absenteeism. *Health Policy and Planning,* 1–10. doi: 10.1093/heapol/czw046..

Ackers, H. L., Ackers-Johnson, J., Chatwin, J., & Tyler, N. (2017). *Healthcare, frugal innovation, and professional voluntarism: A cost-benefit analysis.* New York: Palgrave.

Ackers-Johnson, J. (2010). Internal student benchmarking Report. SVP.

Altbach, P. G., & Knight, J. (2007). The internationalization of higher education: Motivations and realities. *Journal of Studies in International Education,* *11*(3–4), 290–305.

Banerjee, A. (2010). Medical electives: A chance for international health. *Journal of the Royal Society of Medicine, 103,* 6–8.

Bates et al. (2014). *Perspectives on context: A selection of essays considering the role of context in successful quality improvement.* London: The Health Foundation.

© The Author(s) 2017

A. Ahmed et al., *The Ethics of Educational Healthcare Placements in Low and Middle Income Countries,* DOI 10.1007/978-3-319-48363-4

Bourdieu, P., & Passeron, J. C. (1990). *Reproduction in education, society and culture (Vol. 4)*. London: Sage.

British Council. (2013). Annual report. The British Council. London.

British Medical Association. (2009). *Ethics and medical electives in resource-poor countries. A Tool Kit*. London: BMA.

Brookfield, S. (1995). The getting of wisdom: What critically reflective teaching is and why it's important. In Brookfield, S (Ed.), *Becoming a reflective teacher* (pp. 1–28). San Fransisco. Jossey-Bass:

Brooks, R., & Waters, J. (2009). A second chance at 'success' UK students and global circuits of higher education. *Sociology, 43*(6), 1085–1102.

Brooks, R., & Waters, J. (2011). *Student mobilities, migration and the internationalisation of higher education*. Basingstoke: Palgrave Macmillan.

Clampin, A. (2008). Overseas placements: Addressing our challenges. *British Journal of Occupational Therapy, 71*(8), 354–356.

Coates, P. C. (2006). The new medical missionaries – grooming the next generation of global healthworkers. *The English Journal of Medicine, 354*(17), 1771–1773.

Coey, C. (2013). International academics in English higher education: Practicing and capturing mobile careers'. Unpublished PhD thesis. http://repository.liv.ac.uk/17813/

Cox, D. (2008). Evidence of the main factors inhibiting mobility and career development of researchers. Final report to the European commission. Contract DG-RTD-2005-M-02-01. http://ec.europa.eu/euraxess/pdf/research_policies/rindicate_final_report_2008_11_june_08_v4.pdf. Accessed 19 October 2016.

Dasco, M., Chandra, A., & Friedman, H. (2013). Adopting an ethical approach to global health training: The evolution of the Botswana-University of Pennsylvania partnership. *Academic Medicine, 88*(11), 1646–1650.

De Wit, H. (2008). The internationalisation of higher education in global context. In H. De Wit, P. Agarwal, M. F. Said, M. T. Sehoole, & M. Sirozi (Eds.), *The dynamics of international student circulation in a global context*. Rotterdam: Sense Publishers.

Dowell, J., & Merryless, N. (2009). Electives: Isn't it time for a change? *Medical Education, 43*, 121–126.

Drain, P. K., Hunt, D. D., Fawzi, W. W., Homes, K. K., & Gardner, P. (2007). Global health in medical education: A call for more training and opportunities. *Academic Medicine, 82*(3), 226–230.

Elit, L., Hunt, M., Redwood-Campbell, L., Ranford, J., Adelson, N., & Schwartz, L. (2011). Ethical issues encountered by medical students during international health electives. *Medical Education, 45*, 704–711.

Ericsson, K. A., Krampe, R. T., & Tesch-Romer, C. (1993). The role of deliberate practice in the acquisition of expert performance. *Psychological Review, 100*(3), 363–406.

Findlay, A. M., Stam, A., King, R., & Ruiz-Gelices, E. (2005). International opportunities: Searching for the meaning of student migration. *Geogrphaica Helvetica, 60*(3), 192–200.

Francis, R. (2013). *Report of the mid Staffordshire NHS foundation trust public inquiry*. London: HMSO.

Gedde, M., Edjang, S., & Mandeville, K. (2011). *Working in international health*. Oxford: Oxford University Press.

Hanson, L., Harms, S., & Plamondon, K. (2011). Undergraduate international medical electives: Some ethical and pedagogical considerations. *Journal of Studies in International Education, 15*(2), 171–185.

Hastings, A., Dowell, J., & Kalmus Eliasz, A. (2014). Medical student electives and learning outcomes for global health: A commentary on behalf of the UK medical schools elective council. *Medical Teacher, 36*, 355–357.

Horton, A. (2009). Internationalising occupational therapy education. *British Journal of Occupational Therapy, 72*(5), 227–230.

Hudson, S., & Inkson, K. (2006). Volunteer overseas development workers: The hero's adventure and personal transformation. *Career Development International, 11*(4), 304–320.

Huish, R. (2012). The ethical conundrum of international health electives in medical education. *Journal of Global Citizenship & Equity Education, 2*(1), 1–19.

Jeffrey, J., Dumont, R. A., Kim, G. Y., & Kuo, R. (2011). Effects of international health electives on medical student learning and career choice: Results of a systematic literature review. *Family Medicine, 43*(1), 21–28.

Larsen, J., & Jacobsen, M. H. (2009). Metaphors of mobility – inequality on the move. In H. Maksim & M. M. Bergman (Eds.), *Mobilities and inequality* (pp. 75–96). London: Routledge.

Longstaff, B. (2012). *Toolkit for the collection of evidence of knowledge and skills gained through involvement in international health links*. London: Northumbria Healthcare NHS Foundation Trust.

Macfarlane, A. J., & Dorkenoo, E. (2015). *Prevalence of female genital mutilation in England and Wales: National and local estimates*. London: City University London in association with Equality Now.

Mdee, A., & Emmott, R. (2008). Social enterprise with international impact: The case for fair trade certification of volunteer tourism. *Education, Knowledge and Economy, 2*(3), 191–201.

Meyer, J.-B. (2003). 'Policy implications of the brain drain's changing face', SciDevNet: Policy Brief May 2003. Available at: www.scidev.net/dossiers/index.cfm?fuseaction=policybrief&dossier=10&policy=24

Molesworth, M., Scullion, R., & Nixon, E. (2011). *The marketisation of higher education and the student as consumer*. London: Routledge.

Moyo, D. (2009). *Dead aid. Why aid is not working and how there is another way for Africa*. London: Penguin.

Murdoch-Eaton, D., & Green, A. (2011). The contribution and challenges of electives in the development of social accountability in medical students. *Medical Teacher, 33*(8), 643–648.

National Health Service. (2016). NHS workforce statistics, September 2015, England, Experimental. http://content.digital.nhs.uk/catalogue/PUB20335. Accessed 12 October 2016.

National Health Service Digital. (2016). Healthcare workforce statistics, England. NHS digital. http://content.digital.nhs.uk/catalogue/PUB21783/nhs-staf-sep-2015-mar-2016-rep.pdf. Accessed 5 October 2016.

Norton, D., & Marks-Maran, D. (2014). Developing cultural sensitivity and awareness in nursing overseas. *Nursing Standard, 28*(44), 39–43.

Organisation for Economic Cooperation and Development (OECD). (2015). http://www.oecd-ilibrary.org/. Accessed 30 November 2016.

Petrosoniak, A., McCarthy, A., & Varpio, L. (2010). International health electives: Thematic results of student and professional interviews. *Medical Education, 44*, 683–689.

Polonijo-King, I. (2004). In whose words? Narrative analysis of international volunteer stories from an anthropological perspective. *Narodna umjetnost-Hrvatski casopis za etnologiju i folkloristiku, 21*(1), 103–121.

Raphaely, N., & O'Moore, E. (2010). Understanding the health needs of migrants in the South East region. A report by the South East migrant health study group on behalf of the department of health.

Raymond, E. M., & Hall, C. M. (2008). The development of cross-cultural (mis) understanding through volunteer tourism. *Journal of Sustainable Tourism, 16*(5), 530–543.

Regets, M. C. (2003). Impact of skilled migration on receiving countries. SciDevNet Policy Brief, May. Available at: www.scidev.net/dossiers/index.cfm?fuseaction=policybrief&policy=21&dossier=10

Rominksi, S. D., Yakubu, J., Rockefeller, A. O., Peterson, M., Tagoe, N., & Bell, SA. (2015). The role of short term volunteers in a global health capacity building effort: The project HOPE-GEMC experience. *International Journal of Emergency Medicine, 8*, 23.

Royal College of Midwives. (2011). RCM survey of student midwives 2011: UK national survey.

Sharpe, E. K., & Dear, S. (2013). Points of discomfort: Reflections on power and partnerships in international service-learning. *Michigan Journal of Community Service Learning, 19*, 49–57.

Sharpe, V. A. (1997). Why "do no harm"? In D. C. Thomasma (Ed.), *The influence of Edmund D. Pellegrino's philosophy of medicine* (pp. 197–215). the Netherlands: Springer.

Simpson, K. (2004). 'Doing development': The gap year, volunteer-tourists and a popular practice of development. *Journal of International Development, 16,* 681–692.

Snee, H. (2013). Volunteer tourism and the 'cosmopolitan' gap year. *Global Discourse, 4*(1), 44–46.

Stephens, M. (2015). Changing student nurses values, attitudes and behaviours: A meta ethnography of enrichment activities. *Nursing and Care, 5*(1), 320–322.

Topping, J. (2015). Policing in Northern Ireland: Research, meaning and lessons from a contested landscape.

Waugh, A., Smith, D., Horsburgh, D., & Gray, M. (2014). Towards a values-based person specification for recruitment of compassionate nursing and midwifery candidates: A study of registered and student nurses' and midwives' perceptions of prerequisite attributes and key skills. *Nurse Education Today, 34*(9), 1190–1195. doi:10.1016/j.nedt.2013.12.009Francis report 2013.

Wearing, S., & McGehee, N. G. (2013). Volunteer tourism: A review. *Tourism Management, 38,* 120–130.

Williams, A. (2006). Lost in translation? International migration. *Learning and Knowledge Transfer Progress in Human Geography, 30*(5), 588–607.

Williams, A., & Ballaz, V. (2008). Factors shaping intra-European student migration: Understanding knowledge flows.

# INDEX

© The Author(s) 2017
A. Ahmed et al., *The Ethics of Educational Healthcare Placements in Low and Middle Income Countries*, DOI 10.1007/978-3-319-48363-4

Printed in the United States
By Bookmasters